Successful scientific writing

Successful scientific writing is a user-friendly book providing detailed practical guidance to help students and researchers in the biological and medical sciences to communicate their work effectively through the published literature.

This acclaimed step-by-step guide covers all aspects of typescript preparation from first to final draft, including word processor use and electronic database literature services. Abundant examples, practical advice and self-help exercises draw on the authors' extensive experience with actual typescripts. Uniform typescript format conventions given here are accepted by 500+ journals.

Applicable to a variety of scientific writing contexts in the majority of disciplines, *Successful Scientific Writing* is a powerful tool for improving individual skills, as well as an eminently suitable text for classroom courses or seminars on scientific writing.

JANICE R. MATTHEWS, a writer and educator with a broad background in the biological sciences, has edited hundreds of scientific research papers in the veterinary and biological sciences, both in university settings and for private industry. She currently owns and operates Scientific Editing Services in Athens, Georgia.

JOHN M. BOWEN is Emeritus Professor of Pharmacology and Toxicology, former Associate Dean for Research and Graduate Affairs, and former Director of the Veterinary Medical Experiment Station at the University of Georgia.

ROBERT W. MATTHEWS is Professor of Entomology at the University of Georgia where he teaches insect behavior, animal behavior and entomology for teachers. His research specialities are wasps and bees.

The Matthews have worked and written together for over 30 years. Together they have authored eight books and numerous scientific and popular publications. Their current joint enterprise is the WOWBugs Project, an extensive life science curriculum development endeavor.

Successful scientific writing

A step-by-step guide
for the biological
and medical sciences

Second edition

Janice R. Matthews,
John M. Bowen, and
Robert W. Matthews

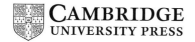
CAMBRIDGE
UNIVERSITY PRESS

PUBLISHED BY THE PRESS SYNDICATE OF THE UNIVERSITY OF CAMBRIDGE
The Pitt Building, Trumpington Street, Cambridge, United Kingdom

CAMBRIDGE UNIVERSITY PRESS
The Edinburgh Building, Cambridge CB2 2RU, UK
40 West 20th Street, New York, NY 10011-4211, USA
477 Williamstown Road, Port Melbourne, VIC 3207, Australia
Ruiz de Alarcón 13, 28014 Madrid, Spain
Dock House, The Waterfront, Cape Town 8001, South Africa

http://www.cambridge.org

First published 1996
Second edition 2000
Reprinted 2001, 2003

Printed in the United Kingdom at the University Press, Cambridge

Typeset in Ehrhardt 10/12pt [VN]

A catalogue record for this book is available from the British Library

Library of Congress Cataloguing in Publication data

Matthews, Janice R., 1943–
Successful scientific writing: a step-by-step guide for the biological and medical
sciences/Janice R. Matthews, John M. Bowen, Robert W. Matthews – 2nd ed.
    p.   cm.
Includes bibliographical references (p.   ).
ISBN 0 521 78962 1 (pb)
1. Medical writing.   I. Bowen, John M.   II. Matthews, Robert W., 1942–
III. Title.
R119.M28 2000
808'.06661–dc21   00-036043

ISBN 0 521 78962 1 paperback

Contents

Preface

Mend your speech a little, lest it mar your fortune.
William Shakespeare

The catch phrase "Publish or Perish" – or its more upbeat variant, "Publish and Flourish" – seems to have as much validity as ever in the minds of scientists everywhere. The scientific community has long emphasized quantity and quality of scholarly publications as a way to judge the eminence of scientists. Granting agencies appear to do the same. Scores received by renewal applications for National Institutes of Health funding for research in universities and hospitals have been shown to correlate very strongly with the number of publications resulting from NIH grants. Perhaps it is not surprising that the publication rate of scientific information doubles about every 12 years (Stix, 1994), although few of us will be likely to match the output of a Russian chemist whose scientific productivity over 10 years totaled 948 papers, or about one publication every 4 days!

All this writing . . . Does it really make any difference whether it is good, bad, or ugly? We believe it does, and that it matters a great deal, for words are tools of science no less than numbers are. Research is not complete until it is communicated, and publication in a refereed journal is the fundamental unit of scientific communication. The decision not only to write, but to make the effort to write well, lies at the heart of scientific literacy. To most minds, sloppy scientific writing indicates sloppy thinking, and both are disastrous to research and research reporting.

The published word has remarkable persistence. A sloppily written or prematurely published paper can haunt a scientist to the end of his or her days. Over 30 years ago, an examination of the reasons why research grant applications were turned down showed that 12% of the rejected proposals were not approved because the investigators' previously published work did not inspire confidence. Despite vast technological advances, there is no reason to expect that scientific writing is any less important today.

Still, we never set out to be writers. Few scientists do. During our graduate training, we learned about statistics, research, experimentation; we were taught to use instruments and techniques we have seldom encountered again. There was never a word of guidance on writing a scientific paper, nor did we notice that this instruction was missing . . . at first. Once our working lives began, we quickly learned that while a plumber can make a comfortable living without writing about his pipes, a scientist's career is inextricably enmeshed with (some would say enslaved by) the need to write. So, like most scientists, we have stumbled along, learning writing skills by trial and error now and then helped along by a benevolent senior faculty member or a friendly colleague.

Now, as a new millennium begins, we find we have become that senior faculty member and, hopefully, those friendly colleagues as well. This guidebook is one outcome. Its goals are to help you to write effectively and efficiently, just as we would if we could meet with you in person. Because it forms such a major part of almost every scientist's written communication, the research article in a biological, medical, or veterinary medical journal is the book's main focus. However, the tips, techniques, and guidelines presented here apply to a variety of other writing contexts, from review articles to the popular press.

The first edition of *Successful scientific writing* began as a brief manual requested by graduate students and new researchers affiliated with the University of Georgia's College of Veterinary Medicine, and their colleagues in human medicine and the biological sciences. This second edition has been reorganized and expanded to offer increased guidance, additional examples, and more hands-on exercises.

When you picked up this book, did you fear that it would center on split infinitives, case and tense, and other matters that sound only too much like English Composition class? They will be covered – but we promise this won't be grammar class revisited. We do not aspire to present you with a comprehensive reference work or stylebook, chock-full of detailed grammatical and stylistic rules and obscure exceptions to them. Where such specialized information might be desirable, we try instead to point you toward relevant resources.

Efficiency and effectiveness include far more than wordsmithing. While good writing seems synonymous with a great deal of revising, rereading, and polishing, we believe that effective scientific writing is not as difficult to accomplish as many people try to make it. We hope to show you how to develop a strong organizational framework for both the task and the document, how to access the literature more effectively, and how to tailor your approach to your individual style. We have shared a potpourri of techniques which have been useful in our own writing – covering aspects as varied as overcoming writer's block, using word processors, and constructing tables and graphs. To illustrate the guidelines and suggestions, we have provided abundant examples and exercises, many of which are based upon actual manuscripts slated for publication in scientific journals in the biological and medical sciences.

Our scientific community is rapidly becoming an international one, and English is becoming a truly global language. New sections in this edition cover using the Internet and email, and special tips when writers and readers have different first languages. Because we are most accustomed to American spelling, grammar, abbreviations, and punctuation, we have usually followed American conventions in these matters. However, we have tried to point out British equivalents or alternatives whenever possible.

Any book can only do so much, especially in as personal an area as writing. Learning to write skillfully is, always has been, and must continue to be a hands-on experience. However, it needn't be the random, slow, haphazard process that typically occurs in academic circles. Whether you use this book as an alternative to a formal course in science communication or to complement such a course, we hope that you will find that studying and applying this material increases your awareness of scientific writing style. Our goal is to help ease your approach to the writing which your chosen profession in the sciences will invariably call upon you to do.

J.R.M.
J.M.B.
R.W.M.

1

From start to finish: the big picture

A naturalist's life would be a happy one if he had only to observe
and never to write.

Charles Darwin

Even the most successful scientists usually would rather conduct new research than write a new draft. Communication is essential to scientific progress, however. As surely as dusk follows dawn, a research project must generate a written publication if it is to have lasting value. This is how science moves forward, with the written word illuminating each step of discovery for the sake of others that follow. By presenting an overview of the entire process, this chapter endeavors to make the journey begin a bit more smoothly.

SCIENTIFIC WRITING BEGINS WHERE RESEARCH DOES – WITH A QUESTION

Scientific writing almost always begins with a question that cannot be definitively answered out of our previous personal experiences. What chemicals make up this attractant pheromone? Why did these patients develop high blood pressure? Where are other members of this species found? The list is as varied and limitless as the complexities of nature.

Any time we reach past our own knowledge and experience to seek out, investigate, and use materials beyond our personal resources, research is involved. It may be the study of a subject through firsthand observation and investigation, such as carrying out a laboratory experiment, conducting a survey, or sifting through statistical data. Or it may be the examination of studies that other researchers have made of a subject, as presented in books, articles, or scientific debates. Most often it is a combination of the two.

The first substantial writing that many beginning scientists produce is a prospectus or progress report on their thesis work or a short journal article written jointly with their supervisor or major professor. In academia, this often is followed by a thesis or dissertation. To encourage early attention to the writing phase of science, an increasing number of major professors, departments, and entire colleges and universities are requesting a detailed prospectus, including a literature review, before granting permission for research projects to begin. Many

1

are also urging or requiring that theses and dissertations be presented in the style of a series of single-topic papers suitable for submission, often concurrently, to various appropriate journals. Some even accept papers published before the dissertation is completed, with reprints being bound into the dissertation.

Literature review and prospectus-writing skills are more than academic, however. In business and industry, not only must a well-written proposal precede approval for research projects, but often it can spell the difference in matters of promotion and pay. In fact, one would be hard pressed to find any scientific profession that would not require checking sources of information about a specific subject, integrating this information with one's own ideas, and presenting thoughts, findings, and conclusions effectively.

A book like this one is not the place for a detailed procedural catalogue of all the profitable ways of doing research. Conducting a comprehensive literature review or a research study is undeniably a big job. Presumably you are being guided through these steps by other mentors. However, we would offer a brief overview of scientific writing, preceded by a few general points of advice to help you coordinate your work.

Keep the big picture in mind

Begin by asking yourself some important questions about your plans for the research itself (Table 1.1). Seek advice on these matters. If necessary, modify your plans accordingly.

Periodically assess research progress and direction

When a study has been under way for a while, it is time to check the direction the work is taking. Force yourself to sit down and describe its progress in writing. The discipline of marshaling words into formal sentences will compel you to think about the work more clearly.

If possible, this is a good time to present your methods and results orally or in poster form at a public forum such as a laboratory meeting, a departmental seminar, or a scientific conference whose proceedings are limited to abstracts. The comments and questions you receive will help you to decide whether you need to do more research and to notice where more work is needed to fill gaps in your arguments and observations.

After these preliminary assessments, it's time to ask a hard question. Is your study really worth writing about? The answer to that big question is yes only if your results and conclusions fulfill one of these requirements:

> They are reasonably consistent, reproducible, and complete.
> They represent significant experimental, theoretical, or observational extensions of knowledge.
> They represent advances in the practical application of known principles.
> They take knowledge of the subject a step further.

Table 1.1. *Preliminary questions to ask about research design*

The basic question	Examples of ways in which it might be assessed
1. Do I know what I'm doing?	Have I drawn up a plan (a protocol) for what I intend to do? Do the proposed studies cover all the criticisms likely to be made? Are the statistical methods valid?
2. Do my proposed experiments meet accepted ethical standards?	If my experiments involve human beings or animals, do they meet accepted standards? Could my work adversely affect the environment or the place where I am doing field work?
3. What practical and political considerations need to be addressed?	Is publication of my work likely to break any official secrecy regulations? Could publication invalidate a later application for a patent?
4. How will I record the work as it proceeds?	How will I record what I read? How will I record what I do? How will I ensure that my records are complete? How will I ensure that I can access the records again when I or others need them?

In other words, are the outcomes of your study new, true, and meaningful? If the answer to all these questions is no, delay publication efforts. Sometimes, a topic that originally looked worthwhile turns out to be a dud or simply unsuitable in its present form. Don't throw away the data, but defer writing a paper based on them until further work has been done. Make it your aim to publish a few first-rate articles rather than numerous second-rate contributions. Poor quality publications can come back to haunt you later.

Organization is a journey, not a destination

Once a question has been identified, a literature review is almost always the first step in scientific research. The review reveals reports of similar work, helps narrow the research question, and suggests appropriate avenues to publication. It also generally results in a lot of paper-shuffling – which makes effective organization an obligation, not an option, for the successful writer.

It is essential to have some system in place to deal with all the information that will be converging upon you. You'll soon be handling an avalanche of papers, from personal notes to photocopies to journal reprints. In addition, some scientific societies are concurrently publishing their journals on the Internet now, and experts predict that many may switch solely to electronic publication in the future (Walker, 1998). Articles in these journals will be viewed, searched, copied to another application, and printed in full or in part.

What system is most effective? There is no one-size-fits-all answer. Every situation requires a slightly different style of organization to get the job done, and people generally perform best with techniques tied to their own per-sonal style and energy level. We find it helpful to set up separate file folder "reservoirs" for each section of the eventual paper before beginning to collect notes. As relevant information appears, we number it, date it, and sort it into these separate files. (Numbering everything makes it easier to refer to when writing a first draft.) As thoughts occur to us, we write them on separate sheets of paper (so there will be room to add to them later if needed) and add these papers to the appropriate reservoirs as well. One of us keeps these notes in a loose-leaf notebook. Another just piles the folders in a box.

The popular press is brimming with suggestions for organizational systems, often coupled with explicit or implicit promises of spectacular life results if one can only become properly organized (e.g., Covey, 1989; Aslett, 1996; Bolker, 1998). Seek out such materials if you feel you need motivation, inspiration, or novel suggestions, but maintain your perspective. The secret to effective and efficient scientific writing isn't simply in getting organized. It's in wanting to get the job done and committing oneself to do it.

Whatever system you choose, start using it promptly and stay up with it consistently. Copy or print out at least the abstract of any potentially helpful article. Do not use these photocopies as a substitute for taking notes, however. Because of the way that writing and thinking are related to each other, attempt to digest these written materials as you go along. Postponing this step until later will only make writing more difficult and prolonged. Instead, adopt a good note-taking procedure right from the start. Take many more notes than you think you need and prune them later. To avoid unintentional plagiarism, always write notes in your own words. If you must break this rule, use extreme care to identify quoted material either with quotation marks or with the letter *Q*.

Use many different search strategies

Trace information in all directions through time and space. Each search strategy has different strengths and weaknesses, and will uncover a somewhat different set of information.

Chapter 2 covers computerized searches in some detail. However, the idea of networking predates computers by a long shot. For example, a time-honored search strategy called the Ancestry Approach starts by acquiring a research report and examining its references to find other relevant references. Through reiteration, researchers work their way back through the literature until either the important concepts disappear or the studies become so old they can be judged obsolete. A newer set of searching tools employs the Descendency Approach. Citation indexes identify a publication's offspring – those more recent books and journal articles that reference the earlier work.

Make it easy to relocate relevant material

Write the full journal source on each photocopy or computer printout, if the source is not printed somewhere on the page. For material obtained from online sources, make a paper ("hard") copy of important information. List the author, if available; title, document, file, or Web site; date of the material; name of the database or other online source; date you accessed the source; and the full electronic address or Uniform Resource Locator (URL; see Chapter 2).

It is particularly easy to forget how one actually located online material. To minimize this problem, it is a good idea to make an electronic bookmark that identifies a location you may want to revisit. Label the bookmark with a term applicable to the associated information source. Over time, these bookmarks will accumulate into a customized list that makes it easy to locate and return to particular sites.

THE MESSAGE DETERMINES THE MEDIUM

Once the literature review is complete and research is underway, it is time to give further consideration to the writing task that is ahead. At this point, a savvy writer asks four questions.

1. What message do I want to convey?
2. Which format is most appropriate for my message?
3. Who will be interested in my message?
4. Where should this paper be published?

You may be able to answer these questions by yourself, but for an extra margin of safety, discuss them with a more experienced colleague. All of us can suffer from the normal human failings of inflating the importance of a message and overestimating the size and nature of its potential audience.

What message do I want to convey?

By this point, you should be able to answer this question in some detail. In essence, it can be rephrased as: "What is my research question, and what is (or probably will be) my answer?"

This is not the same as asking the "purpose" of the research. That phrasing can lead to some tremendously circular and meaningless statements: "The purpose of my research was to obtain data so I could publish them in order to get my degree so I could do more research and publish some more . . ."

Which format is most appropriate for my message?

Most of us are justifiably interested in recognition for our work. The way in which a study is formatted and published can determine the nature of that recognition, and in fact whether we receive any recognition at all.

For a scientist to receive professional credit for being the first to discover something new, it is not sufficient just to be the first to perceive or detect it – he or she must be the first to publish the information "validly," i.e., in a very specific way. This distinction is most important in (but not restricted to) the taxonomic sciences, in which the naming of new organisms hinges on a strict system of priority of valid publication.

"Valid" scientific publication has several essential components. It is (1) the first publication of research results (2) in a form whereby peers can repeat the experiment and test its conclusions, (3) appearing in a primary journal or other source document (4) that is readily available within the scientific community. In addition, (5) the scientific paper contains certain specified kinds of information (6) organized in a certain stylized manner, i.e., it has a certain format. This is not to imply that other publication is "invalid" for any other use than this very special purpose of establishing priority of discovery.

Though they may be designated by slightly different sets of names, research papers in the biological and medical sciences fall into four general categories – research articles, case histories, reviews, and case-series analyses – and shorter variants with such titles as research notes or brief communications. Each category is most appropriate for different sorts of messages.

Research articles and case histories are the usual avenue for valid publication of original results. Both types of papers are based on one's own experiences. A research article generally presents new data obtained through experimentation or observation. A case history usually covers such subjects as a unique, previously undescribed syndrome or disease, new information on an illness, an unsuspected causal relationship, or an unexpected outcome such as a possible therapeutic or adverse drug effect. The study may be retrospective (analyzing previously accumulated data) or prospective (with a design that predates data collection).

Satisfying a requirement for valid publication, research articles and case histories have a specific set of defining characteristics. Both are structured with distinctive sections that parallel the sequence of a critical argument. They present a question (sometimes formally stated as a hypothesis). They marshal evidence to support various possible answers to the question. Finally, they attempt to persuade the reader of the truth of a particular choice of answers.

Review articles and case-series analyses, on the other hand, cover principally other scientists' discoveries rather than one's own. This is not to downplay their importance, nor to suggest that they are in any way "invalid" or second-rate. Reviews, such as those found in the *Annual Review of . . .* series, perform a valuable role by synthesizing the results of a search through literature or other records. They often are heavily relied on by someone entering a subject for the first time and for communication between scientists. They can also introduce new ways of looking at a topic, and point out flaws or gaps in scientific understanding or in the published literature.

The structure and format of reviews and other summary analyses are less standardized than those of a research article. If there is a "methods" section, it often states the manner and extent of the search. If a series of cases is being included, it often tells what records were accessed. The organizational sequence of these papers depends on the topic. Commonly, items are covered either in chronological order, from general to particular, or from frequent occurrence to rare. Both reviews and case-series analyses may yield new insights, hypotheses, and understanding, and in that sense they also constitute "valid" original research.

In addition to research articles and case series, shorter variants have arisen, which address the need for quicker, but less comprehensive transmission of results. These may be called by such titles as research notes, short communications, or research briefs.

What is a "primary journal or other source document that is readily available within the scientific community"? Primary and secondary has nothing to do with quality or importance. Rather, a primary journal is merely one that details firsthand information reported by people directly involved with an action or event. A secondary journal presents information that does not come directly from people involved in the action or event. Rather, it is reported by a second (or third) person removed from the source. Some of these publications, such as the Elsevier journals, are significant sources of communication among scientists and the educated public, particularly with the increased availability which the Internet provides. See, for example, *Trends in Cell Biology* <www.biomednet.com/library/tcb>.

Popular articles – secondary accounts designed to entertain as well as to inform – may not adhere to the rigorous standards of regular scientific articles. They typically offer only a condensed overview of the methodology used and a summary of the major findings, without presenting actual data. For these reasons, popular articles do not generally constitute valid publication. However, writing or providing consultation for popular articles based on validly published scientific research should be an important part of a scientist's outreach activities to the wider community that supports his or her work.

Who will be most interested in my message?

Most of us have pretty healthy egos. We think our writing will merit the attention of far more readers than it will in fact attract. This nearly universal failing can lead to poor choice of a potential journal, and this poor choice can lead to delays, requests for major revision, or outright rejection.

Two closely related, bluntly asked questions can help a writer find the most appropriate audience.

> *So what?* This question could be cast less abruptly in any of several ways. What effect will my message have on concepts or practices? Why should readers pay attention to it? Will it lead to widespread changes in the way we view the world?
>
> *Who cares?* One could also ask this question more mildly. Who will be the most interested in this information? Will it be the specialists in a small field? Or most practitioners? Or the scientific world in general?

Be realistic. Don't get caught up in contemplating a vast potential audience that "needs" to know your information. In this information-filled world, no one should be expected to make brain-room for data simply because the facts are currently unknown to him or her. The more accurately one can answer these questions, the more precise one's journal publication options become.

And the more precisely one targets a journal, the better the chances for publication.

Where should this paper be published?

Even within a single specialized area, journals differ in such vital aspects as topic coverage, format, speed of publication, acceptance rate, page charges, and presumed prestige. Their readership varies as well. For the greatest efficiency and the best chance of acceptance and prompt publication, search early and well for the best match of topic, journal, and audience you can possibly achieve.

Refer to those abstracting services or indexes (see Chapter 2) that you used to begin a literature search and use them to help identify potential avenues for publication. Did your literature search indicate that one or more journals were the principal sources of reports related to your research? Examine current issues of periodicals in which others in your field have published. Note that some journals with scientific society sponsorship may require that an author or coauthor be a society member.

If you are really unsure what your choices are, begin by getting more information about journals in your field (Table 1.2). Colleagues and librarians are two logical sources of information. Compilations of *Instructions to Authors (ITAs)* such as the *Author's Guide to Biomedical Journals* (Anonymous, 1994) and Atlas (1995) can help you compare the focus, objectives, and submission requirements for a large number of journals.

Evaluate journal suitability and impact

After identifying a few promising possibilities, go to the library and scan some recent issues. Check the table of contents. Look inside the front or back cover. Nearly all will have two items of special interest – a statement of the journal's scope, and a variably titled set of editorial guidelines we've chosen to call *Instructions to Authors* or *ITAs*. Do they seem appropriate for the topic and type of paper you will be preparing?

Generally, if a journal is regularly publishing a number of papers on topics similar to yours, you stand a better chance of acceptance than if very few papers related to your topic have appeared. However, stay open to considering journals outside your field. Editors today increasingly seem to be accepting papers on the basis of their importance to the journal's audience, rather than on the basis of narrowly defined academic fields. If you feel your topic would be of more than peripheral interest to the journal's audience, it is quite appropriate to query the editor.

Will your colleagues still see your paper if you publish it here? One way to determine whether scientists in your field are reading this journal is to examine the "Cited Journal Package" in *Journal Citation Reports* (see Table 2.2 on pages 28–29). This helpful feature gives the number of citations of a given journal's papers in other journals during a calendar year. The list is subdivided to show which journals have carried those citations and how many appeared in each.

Table 1.2. *Sample questions to ask when considering a journal for potential publication of a scientific research paper*

1. What type of journal is it?
2. Is the topic of my proposed paper within the journal's scope?
3. Is the topic represented in the journal frequently or only rarely?
4. What is the size and type of the journal's audience?
5. What is the journal's rejection rate?
6. What formats are acceptable to the journal?
7. How long does this journal take to publish papers? (How much is editing phase? How much is production phase?)
8. What is the quality of photographic (half-tones) and graphics reproductions?

There is little doubt that the scientific community views journals as having various degrees of "prestige." Like beauty, much of this may lie in the eye of the beholder, for despite repeated efforts, this has been a difficult matter to assess reliably. It certainly is not simply a matter of circulation, for some journals with a high impact on the scientific community have relatively small circulation. *Journal Citation Reports* ranks journals by their relative "impact factors." The impact factor of a given journal is calculated as the number of citations in a given year to papers published in that journal in the preceding 2 years, divided by the number of papers the journal published in that same 2-year period. Comparing the impact factors for journals in a particular field can give a sort of "reality check" in the form of a quantitative clue as to their relative intellectual influence.

A caveat is in order here. Most of us would like to think that the best choice for each of our publications would be a prestigious large-circulation journal. We pretty well know which these are in our field, and we would love to build our reputation by publishing in them. This is normal. However, remember that the match of topic, journal, and audience is the critical issue. Only if a topic really and truly is so revolutionary and of such potential impact that its match with one of these journals seems perfect, should one feel compelled to seek out one of these high-profile journals. High-prestige journals have high rejection rates. Because many receive between 1000 and 4000 typescripts per year, their rejection rates may run as high as 90%. Subjecting a paper to these lottery-like odds means a fairly sizable risk of living in limbo for weeks (and probably months), only to ultimately receive a rejection notice.

If after conscientiously going through all of these steps, you still feel unsure whether you have picked the right journal and the right format, it is acceptable to email, write, or call the editor and raise the question. Frame your query diplomatically. Don't ask, "Will you publish my . . .?" or "Will you publish a review of the diagnosis and treatment of . . .?" Instead, ask "Are you willing to consider for publication a 50-page detailed review of the diagnosis and treatment of . . .?" You may learn that the editor has just accepted such a review, or that the journal never publishes reviews that long – a disappointment for the moment, but an answer that can save you time and work.

If information regarding publication time is not indicated in *Instructions to Authors*, it is also appropriate to query the editor about this matter, requesting average and range of time from submission to publication. Most editors take pride in their continued efforts to try to reduce the time from submission to publication.

If you are still not sure where your document will ultimately be sent, prepare the typescript according to the requirements outlined in Appendix 2, while continuing to consider journal possibilities. When you make your decision, check the *ITAs* to see whether they specify acceptance of the Uniform Requirements.

Avoid salami-slicing science

One final caveat. As your search begins to uncover a variety of specialized journals, each may seem perfectly suited for reporting a different part of your data. Some studies do justify more than one report, particularly when different portions have given rise to differing messages of interest to different audiences. However, given the importance of publication in academic circles, one often can be tempted to carve clearly related aspects of a study arbitrarily into more documents than is really sensible. When all of the findings together yield a single message that can be presented in a paper of normal length for the intended journal, they belong together. There is no reasonable justification for what one writer (Lawrence, 1981) has called salami science. (We would add that it tends to produce baloney!)

WRITE AND REVISE SYSTEMATICALLY

Has this ever happened to you? Under pressure of a deadline, you must write a paper, but you just can't quite get started and aren't sure quite where to begin anyway. Days pass, and your guilt climbs. Finally, a couple of days before the deadline, your adrenaline kicks in . . . you throw words together in whatever way you can, writing into the wee hours of the morning, then print a copy and hurriedly send it off or turn it in. Not your best effort, you mutter, but considering how little time you had, not too bad, either!

This is an old, sad story. We all have fooled ourselves like this at times. We know in the back of our minds that some time spent on revision would have improved that hastily written paper immensely. But . . . it might take more work, and we're not even quite sure where to begin. What if fiddling around just made the paper worse? What if we ran out of time half-way through? What if . . .? Maybe it would be easier to keep on making excuses.

Take charge with the Process Approach

There is a way to win new control over your writing. It's called the Process Approach. A process is a directed activity in which something changes. Something is always happening – work is being done, a product is being formed, an end of some kind is being achieved. To describe or organize a process, you must

---

Exercise 1–1. Message, format, and audience

How would you answer these questions? Our suggested replies appear in Appendix 1.

1. A 75-year-old woman brought to your clinic has contracted a rare form of viral infection previously known to be associated primarily with children. A quick library search shows that the oldest affected person in the published literature was 62 years old. Should you publish your new information?

2. Your supervisor suggests that you both review the records of the last 50 cases of canine heartworm disease referred to your clinic and coauthor a paper on the findings. You ask what question the paper is going to answer. He is not trying to answer a question, he says irritably. He just wants to report a summary of these data because colleagues elsewhere will be interested. Does the paper have a purpose? Does it have a message? What format would be most appropriate?

3. The two of you go ahead and analyze those 50 cases of heartworm disease. Your analysis doesn't yield any new important findings, but does lend additional support to some previously published views. Is it still publishable? If so, in what form?

4. You've written a concise, clearly worded summary of the genetics of horn development in jackalopes. A series of examples from the literature, combined with your own laboratory analyses and a field-based population study, all point to the conclusion that a single gene controls this trait. You reason that geneticists, veterinary pathologists, and wildlife biologists all should know this important new information. How many papers could justifiably arise from your study?

5. You've gone back through psychiatric clinic records for the past 18 years, and made a startling discovery. Nearly 80% of all the children hospitalized for manic depression had been previously identified in school tests as being highly creative. Who might be the potential audience for your message?

---

analyze its stages. Applied to writing, the Process Approach simply involves methodically breaking the task into discrete stages, and tackling each stage in the most systematic, efficient, and effective way you can determine. We believe that this way of approaching the task will make the writing process more efficient, effective, satisfying, and perhaps even enjoyable, compared with your previous scientific writing efforts.

You have already met the initial step in the process – planning, gathering, and organizing information; Chapter 2 presents additional guidelines for this. Writing the first draft comes next. This stage starts with a number of prewriting steps that are more crucial than most people realize. It includes organizing thoughts with outlines or bubble-charts, and developing tables and figures. Then the first "real" writing begins. We recommend that you write the first draft of the text as continuously as possible, without stopping to fine-tune anything, and then set it aside for a bit.

Revision, an essential part of the process, follows. During the course of writing a first draft, most of us include things in one place which should be in another. One reason for this is that thinking, planning, writing, and revision are not separate processes, since writing is an aid to thinking. Even after careful planning, we think of things as we write. We use words as they come to mind, but our first thoughts are not necessarily the best and they may not be arranged in the most effective order. However, because thinking and writing interact, when the writing task is complete, our understanding of the subject will have been improved.

Although word processing has softened the distinction between writing and editing drafts, it still is helpful to think of the revision process as a series of tasks of successively smaller scale. The first revision concentrates entirely on organization and logic; the second, on broad matters of wording and style; the third, on fine points of grammar, punctuation, and such.

Know when to stop

Writing is only one part of a scientist's work. There comes a time when the task of revision has to stop. Apply cost–benefit analysis to your work. A well-known maxim that seems to apply to a great many endeavors, including revision, states that 20% of the effort is responsible for 80% of the results, and the remaining 80% of the effort only produces an additional 20% of the results.

Revision can be taken too far. We knew a successful artist who would occasionally become so possessed by the urge to "touch up flaws" that we learned to hide the brushes so she couldn't completely obliterate her artwork! Be careful that you do not become so obsessive that the natural flow of your words is lost. Language that is artificial in its bluntness and simplicity may lack interest and style. This is a potential danger of style-analysis computer programs. Blindly taking every suggestion can lead to writing as artificial and stilted as the worst examples of current scientific prose.

Keep tasks in perspective

Each of the chapters in this book presents suggestions and guidelines for dealing efficiently with another of these sequential stages. However, along the way, even a relatively brief handbook like this one presents what can seem like an overwhelming myriad of details. A checklist (Table 1.3) may help keep you from

Table 1.3. *A checklist of the main steps in preparing a research paper for publication*

Action step	Where to find information
Do the primary and/or secondary research necessary to address the research question.	Chapter 2
Assess readiness and direction of the work.	Chapter 1
Choose a probable journal; obtain *Instructions to Authors* and read them; copy examples of tables, figures, and references.	Chapter 1, Chapter 3
Write a working title and choose the main headings.	Chapter 3
Construct concept maps, issue trees, outlines, or other organizational schemes.	Chapter 3
Write the first draft.	Chapter 3
Prepare a preliminary reference list.	Chapter 3
Set the draft aside to give better perspective at revision stage.	Chapter 3
Choose and design tables and figures.	Chapter 4
Revise structure.	Chapter 5
Revise style.	Chapter 5
Revise for word choice.	Chapter 6
Check the grammar.	Chapter 7
Check punctuation and other mechanical matters.	Chapter 8
Obtain comments from colleagues and revise again.	Chapter 1
Obtain permissions to reproduce any previously published materials used.	Chapter 1
Reread *Instructions to Authors* and give the document a final check for format, completeness, and spelling.	Chapter 1, Appendix 2
Prepare final reference listing in proper format, cross-checking all entries with text.	Chapter 1, Appendix 2

losing sight of the forest among the trees. Consider photocopying the checklist, and adding additional columns with target dates for finishing each step and dates of their actual completion.

Important as they may be, don't let the mechanics of writing the paper overbalance the intellectual challenge of pursuing a question that truly interests you and analyzing the science that forms the basis of your research. The excitement of pursuing, developing, and expressing ideas is one of the finest satisfactions of research and scholarship.

ATTENTION TO DETAIL: THE "FINAL" COPY

> Poor spellers of the world, untie!
> *Graffito*

It's two o'clock in the morning. You've just finished going through your document for what seems like the hundredth time. You can no longer really read the words coherently; you only see yourself mechanically reading them. This is the tedious phase, but you can't let up.

Some writers work hard on the first few drafts, then let up their efforts before they complete the final draft. Don't be among that group. Small mistakes at this point will unsettle your reviewers and editor, and will undercut the authority of your work.

Recheck journal format

Long before now you have, of course, chosen a journal. Now it is time to be certain that you have tailored your submission to that journal's requirements. Check the January issue for the journal's current year of publication. There you should find *Instructions for Authors* spelled out. Note, however, that journal *ITAs* vary widely in their comprehensiveness. As you work, you may also need to refer to the "Uniform Requirements for Manuscripts Submitted to Biomedical Journals" reproduced in Appendix 2.

Examine a recent issue for editorial style. Pay attention to the nitty-gritty of matters such as reference citation style, headings and subheadings, use of footnotes, and figure design. Remember that however attractive your pages may look, they are wrong if they are not in the proper format for the publication to which they are being submitted.

Standard practice dictates that typewritten copy should appear in Pica or Elite type, and the spirit of this requirement has carried forward into electronic manuscript preparation. Although computer-generated fonts differ from one another in size, typewritten Pica and Elite type are roughly equivalent to 12-point and 10-point computer-generated type, respectively.

With word processing, select 12-point type and full double (not line-and-a-half) spacing. This is not the time to scrimp on paper. Double space everything that is typed, including tables, figure legends, and footnotes. Use wide margins (a full inch at sides, and at least an inch at top and bottom). Do not even consider reducing the font size to squeeze within a journal's page limitations artificially. Such an attempt at deviousness will only alienate the editors whose approval is critical to the paper's acceptance, and it will probably result in the paper's prompt return.

Mainstream type fonts are of two basic styles, serif and sans serif. A serif is one of the fine cross lines at the bottom or top of a letter such as *I*. Serif fonts have these crossbars; sans serif fonts do not. Type also comes in two types of dimensional spacing, monospace and variable width (proportional). With mono-space fonts such as Courier, every letter occupies the same amount of space, just as they do on a conventional typewriter. Proportional typefaces have letters of varying widths. Unless the *ITAs* specify otherwise, use a proportional serif font style such as New York or Times for the basic text in a conventionally published journal. (Sometimes, a sans serif font such as Courier or Helvetica is used to differentiate tabular material, computer addresses, or other such inclusions.) Electronic journals may use only sans serif fonts.

Even though tables are sometimes printed in smaller type than the text in a journal, the typesetter begins with normal-sized copy. Unless a journal specifically approves it, do not send tables which have been reduced in size on a photocopier. Some journals will permit use of 8.5-inch by 14-inch paper for tables.

On the first page, put the title and author name(s), institutional affiliation(s), corresponding address, telephone and fax numbers, and email address. Often a word count and a suggested running head (short title) are included here as well. The Abstract or Summary appears by itself on the second page. Note whether keywords for indexing services appear here in recent issues of the journal. Mimic the style used.

Begin the Introduction on the third page. Either run the text matter continuously or start each subsequent major section on a separate page. Many journals require the latter approach. Footnotes to text material, if used, are grouped on a separate page, as are figure legends. Each table should each be on a separate page. Rather than interspersing these nontextual materials throughout the text, assemble all of them in numerical order at the back of the typescript. Some journals require notations within the text margins to indicate approximate locations for tables and figures.

Number all pages

In a conventionally typewritten paper, omitting page numbers was a tempting shortcut, because it allowed material to be inserted or changed later without retyping the entire document. Use of a word processor removes this excuse. Given the proper formatting directive, it will automatically repaginate subsequent versions. However, starting major sections on separate pages still can help to minimize reprinting.

Once a typescript begins to pass through the hands of reviewers and editors, page numbers provide the only clues as to whether it has remained complete. Furthermore, these editors and reviewers must be able to refer to pages by number in their written comments. Always number all pages, including (generally in this order) the title page, abstract, the text itself, and such materials as references, tables, figure legends, and footnote lists.

Double-check the accuracy of references and attributions

Several studies of the accuracy of citations and presentations of others' assertions in the biomedical literature have revealed surprisingly high rates of error. An analysis of 300 randomly selected references in six frequently cited veterinary journals found major errors in 30% of them (Hinchcliff *et al.*, 1993). Misquotation rates of 12% in medical journals (deLacey *et al.*, 1985) and 27% in surgical journals (Evans *et al.*, 1990) have been reported.

The most common errors were misspellings, a particularly important problem because they have the potential to impede computerized retrieval systems or obscure author identity. Another common error was a failure to cite the original source of information, a disturbing finding because it suggests that authors frequently do not read the original reference. Misquotations of findings in studies by others also were common, carrying the risk that through repeated secondary citation, a major inaccuracy may become established as accepted fact.

Make it an absolute policy never to try to save time by copying references from someone else's list. Such shortcuts may seem harmless, but it is amazing how easily inaccuracies can creep into reference citations (Blanchard, 1974).

Give the paper its final in-house double review

When the typescript finally seems done, read it once more. Have coauthors or a colleague read it as well. It will undoubtedly still harbor a surprising number of "gremlins." Finding them now is a bit embarrassing, but less so than facing them on the journal reviewer's edited copy or the published page! Make whatever final changes are needed, then print a truly final version to send off.

SUBMIT THE TYPESCRIPT FOR PUBLICATION

No matter what format typescript submission takes, a few basic considerations facilitate matters. The same levels of care and attention to detail that were expended on earlier stages of typescript preparation are needed now. Do not become careless at this point!

Typescript, computer file, or both?

Increasingly, journal editors are encouraging electronic submissions on diskettes or through modem transfer in addition to paper copy. Some journals welcome electronic copy from the beginning. Others delay a request for electronic submission until the modifications based on the review process have been incorporated into the document.

Consult the journal's published *Instructions to Authors* for guidelines on electronic submission. Files prepared using common word processing programs are usually acceptable, but some journals may require that files be converted into ASCII format – plain text without any word processor codes for bold, italics, underlining, subscript, superscript, or unusual or accented characters.

Electronic submission saves editors and publishers time and expense. Editors can edit the typescript on the computer screen, and, if necessary, reformat it to their specific printing requirements. An added advantage is that they can send your article directly to data banks which then store this electronic typescript so that it can be accessed by online systems.

Include a cover letter with the typescript

Write and edit this letter carefully, for it forms an editor's first impression of an author and his or her work. Be certain to spell the editor's name correctly.

Assure that this information is current and correct. Sending a typescript to the wrong person can delay it considerably!

In the letter, name the journal and say something nice (but not effusive) about why it is the appropriate place to publish this particular paper. Mention the title of the typescript, and include your full current address and phone number as corresponding author, in case the letter and typescript should somehow become separated.

When relevant, each of the following points should also be expressly mentioned:

> State that all authors have contributed significantly to the paper, understand and endorse it, and have read and approved the version being submitted for publication. Some journals require a special statement to this effect, signed by all the coauthors; their *ITAs* may specify its wording.
>
> Include a signed permission statement from anyone you've mentioned in the acknowledgments and anyone cited under "personal communication" for use of their name and/or data.
>
> Certify that no part has been submitted, accepted for publication, or published elsewhere.
>
> State that the article is original work of the authors except for material in the public domain or excerpts from others' works for which written permission of the copyright owners has been obtained.
>
> Indicate that the authors have no relationship, financial or otherwise, with any manufacturers or distributors of products evaluated in the paper; if this is not true, disclose any such relationship in a footnote to the paper.
>
> If the paper depends critically on another unpublished paper or one that is "in press" in another journal, mention this fact. Include three copies of the related paper for the reviewers.
>
> Include a statement expressly transferring copyright in the event the paper is published in the journal. All authors must sign this statement. Author(s) may request permission in writing to reuse the document or portions of it.

Also include in the cover letter any additional information that may facilitate editorial processing, such as the type of article (short communication, research article, case study, etc.). It is quite appropriate to offer suggestions for potential nonlocal reviewers.

Make at least three copies, and label everything

Most journals require at least two copies of the typescript, including any supporting materials such as photographs. (Again, check the *Instructions to Authors*.) Save one additional copy for yourself – never mail the sole existing copy of anything! Maintain a backup copy of the final electronic file on a clearly labeled diskette.

Remember Murphy's Law? Anything that can go wrong will, and at the worst possible moment. Assume that packages will become lost in the mail, that photographs will become separated from text, and that figures will be misplaced. Be especially careful to fully label the illustrations, usually done with a sticker label on the reverse side. Note which edge of the illustration is the top. Illustrations are processed differently than text at the publishers, and if unlabeled, proper association of figures and text in the final assembly of the journal can be a headache or worse.

Package it carefully and mail it correctly

Enclose the cover letter and typescript copies in a strong oversized envelope or reinforced mailing bag. If necessary, add a piece of light cardboard to stiffen the package further. Put illustrations and photographs in a separate smaller envelope inside the mailer to protect them further. Place the diskette in a special mailing envelope, and affix it to a page-sized piece of light cardboard to keep it from sliding about during the mailing. When everything is together, seal the mailer and put a strip of tape over the clasp that holds it closed.

When sending a typescript by mail, mark the envelope "First Class Mail" (or "Air Mail" for overseas) very prominently on both the front and back. Otherwise, the postal service may treat it to a much slower third-class mail delivery. Never guess at the proper postage! Take it to a mailroom and have it weighed. For extra speed and security, you may wish to use Priority Mail or a private courier service and request a return receipt.

Now find something else to do. Soon, the journal office may notify you that they have received your submission, but it will be weeks before you hear more than that.

BACK AND FORTH: EDITORIAL REVIEW

Receipt by the editor marks the beginning of a whole series of steps which conclude with publication in printed or electronic media or both. Only two of these steps require direct action from the author: dealing with reviewers' comments and correcting proofs. However, understanding what happens once the editor receives your typescript can help to alleviate those natural feelings of worry and wondering that can gnaw at you while you await a response.

What happens at the editor's office: round one

When it arrives at the editorial office, your typescript is logged in, dated, and assigned a typescript number which allows the editor to track its progress through the subsequent steps. The typescript is also given a cursory review at this stage to assure that all the illustrations are included and that it meets the journal's criteria for submission for publication. The editor then identifies two or three external referees qualified to review your typescript, and sends copies of your typescript to each.

B.C.   **BY JOHNNY HART**

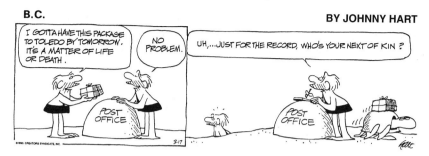

© By permission of Johnny Hart and Creators Syndicate, Inc.

Referees usually are requested to return their reviews within 3 weeks. In an ideal world, all referees would return their reviews promptly, because "peer reviewers" usually are researchers who submit their own work to the same journal and generally they are impatient if they do not receive their own reviews in a timely manner. However, because reviewers volunteer their time, some are less conscientious than others about meeting return deadlines.

Once the editor has all of the external reviews in hand, he or she decides if the paper should be accepted or rejected. The paper then is returned to the corresponding author with copies of the referees' comments and the editor's decision and recommendations.

If the submission is rejected, the author has the option of appealing the decision to the editor or editorial board. Alternatively, the author can choose to reformat the article, incorporate whatever of the reviewer's and editor's recommendations seem warranted, and submit the typescript to another journal, thereby beginning the publication process anew.

Acceptance is nearly always contingent on some revision. Be prepared for this fact. Treat the entire process with respect. As noted by Dizon and Rosenberg (1990), "The peer review process is not a perfect system – just a necessary one."

Deal respectfully with reviewers' comments

The system of peer review, wherein anonymous reviewers funnel comments about your typescript back to you through the editor, is rarely a wholly pleasant one no matter how common it is. Even if you have carefully followed all of the suggestions in this book, be prepared for the possibility of negative reviewer comments.

The worst thing that you can do, should critical reviews appear, is to treat them as an affront to your professional image. Instead, calmly and carefully evaluate all the comments received, point by point. Make the suggested changes that seem to have value. Review those that seem wrong. If a reviewer misunderstood you, try to determine why. The misunderstanding may reveal a weakness in your argument or analysis, or a spot where the writing is weak.

Return the revised typescript to the editor, accompanied by electronic copy if requested. In your letter of reply to the editor, respond to each comment in turn.

Indicate acceptance of those suggestions that seem to have merit. If you chose not to accept a reviewer's comment, indicate why not. Diplomatically and briefly explain your reasoning concerning suggested changes that you feel are unjustified. Avoid anger and any tendency to sarcasm in your responses. Editors sometimes pass your comments back to the reviewer, to whom you may not be anonymous. The world is really a very small place.

What happens at the editor's office: round two

If an author's revisions have been extensive or have substantially changed the paper, the editor may elect to repeat the review process, essentially returning to round one. Once the revised paper is fully acceptable, the editor marks the copy for the typesetter to conform to the particular details of journal design and format. Then the editor forwards it to the publisher.

The publisher typesets the paper and returns it and a galley proof to the author, sometimes by way of the journal's editor, who may also check the proof. Various other paperwork may also appear at this time. Generally the publisher includes an order form for the author to order reprints of the article. If page charges are journal policy, the author receives a bill or invoice for the number of printed pages with the galley proof. Many journals require authors to execute a copyright release form, and such forms are often also enclosed with the galley. In addition to your signature as corresponding author, they may need to be signed by all coauthors.

CORRECT GALLEY PROOF CONSCIENTIOUSLY

"Galley proof" originally was the name for a typeset copy of a document used to permit correction of errors before the type was made up in pages; its name comes from the galley, a tray for holding composed type. With computerized typesetting, the term is also used as a synonym for "page proof" that shows how the made-up pages will appear.

Checking galley proof is an important step in the publication process. Take it seriously, and give the galley the attention and care it deserves. With the increase in electronic submissions, fewer errors are being introduced by the typesetting process, but galleys without errors are exceedingly rare.

Read the proof carefully

Examine individual sentences slowly, word by word and line by line. To detect spelling errors, try reading lines backward to view each word separately. Compare the typeset material with the original typescript to ensure that no material has been omitted or repeated. Examine numbers carefully, especially in tables.

Errors at this stage can be difficult to catch when working alone. If possible, enlist a friend's aid, so that one person can slowly read the original typescript aloud while the other checks the galley.

Mark In Margin	Instruction	Manuscript mark	Corrected type
ℓ	Delete	Science ~~Citation~~ index	Science Index
equine	Insert	the ʌcollarbone	the equine collarbone
(cap)	Capitalize	science citation index	Science Citation Index
(lc)	Make lower case	the Ɇminent biologist	the eminent biologist
(ital)	Italicize	Pseudomonas	*Pseudomonas*
(rom)	Set in roman type	(Muscid)flies	Muscid flies
(bf)	Set in boldface	Methods	**Methods**
(lf)	Set in lightface (no bold)	Dr.(Jones) reported	Dr. Jones reported
⌒	Close up the space	Ma terials	Materials
#	Insert space	Results⌣and⌣Discussion	Results and Discussion
¶	Start a new paragraph	... is new. ʌHowever	... is new. However
(run in)	No paragraph	This finding is new.⌐ ⌐However...	... is new. However...
⊙	Insert a period	Brevity is the key/Try to be simple.	Brevity is the key. Try to be simple.
ʌ/ʌ	Insert the punctuation shown within the carat	Yesʌthe time has comeʌ we are prepared.	Yes, the time has come; we are prepared.

Fig. 1.1. Example of commonly used proofreaders' symbols. Less common proofreading marks can be found in many style manuals, if needed.

Mark corrections attentively

Common sense suggests that a standard method of marking corrections will reduce the chances of misunderstandings. Proofreaders' marks (Fig. 1.1) form an internationally recognized convention, although British and American systems differ slightly. With the galley, publishers may include a list of preferred marks. Common corrections are given in Figure 1.1; for those less commonly used, see O'Connor (1986) and style manuals such as *Scientific Style and Format* (Council of Biology Editors, 1994).

The most frequent corrections are additions and deletions and changes in capitalization, typeface, word order, punctuation, and number style. Mark corrections in the margin and put proofreaders' marks in the body of the text where the errors occur. (Some journals request use of different ink colors for different types of corrections.) Never write the correction itself above the lines of type within the printed matter, as you might with a manuscript or typescript.

Checking over a galley, the printer looks for marginal notations, and makes only the alterations noted there. He or she will not, and cannot be expected to, make sweeping corrections on the basis of a single command such as "change this word to italics throughout the document." Mark each change on the proof where it occurs. When more than one correction must be written in the margin next to a single line of type, arrange them in sequence from left to right, and separate them by slashes (slant lines).

Return proofs promptly

Galley proofs are extremely time-sensitive from the publisher's standpoint. Read and correct the proof and return it immediately to the editor. Delays at this point are costly to everyone.

The time for revision or adding new information has passed. Changes in the typescript at this point should only be to correct errors. Resist any impulse to further polish style. In fact, such changes are usually expressly forbidden, and any changes made that are not the fault of the typesetter may be charged to the author as "penalty copy" at considerable expense. (Rarely, a journal will allow a brief appendix to be added that notes new information that supports work in the paper.)

Enjoy the fruits of your labor

As the final step in the publication process, the editor organizes and makes up an issue from proofed papers, and sends the entire issue to the publisher. The publisher then prints and mails the issue to journal subscribers. Reprints are usually mailed to authors within a week or two of publication.

Now you can at last rejoice! With pride, add this title credit to your growing résumé and begin your next publication.

2

Scientific writing in the computer age

My computer is down. I hope it's something serious.

Graffito

The personal computer has revolutionized scientific writing. Access to a vast interconnected web of information without leaving one's desk is now routine. Communication with far-flung colleagues is virtually instantaneous. Computers have enabled literature databases to be more diverse, comprehensive, and accessible than ever before. Word processing programs have become incredibly sophisticated. One of their advantages is the way in which they have simplified the process of producing clean copies of revised text.

CONDUCT AN EFFICIENT AND THOROUGH LITERATURE SEARCH

It would be a rare research project that did not build in some way upon previous work. How does a researcher go about finding studies relevant to a topic? The answer is different than it was even 10 years ago.

A decade ago, most literature searching was done manually. Computerized literature bases were searchable only when mounted on a mainframe, searching software was difficult to use, and online searching was expensive and limited in scope. Specially trained librarians did most of the searching, and researchers paid telecommunication charges for reaching the mainframe and were charged for each record received.

Today, while the older forms of literature search still have advantages for some purposes, the way in which we obtain information is changing rapidly. In some fields, a literature search that once took six months to a year can often be done in less than 10 minutes, and with far more thorough results. Thousands of specialized databases are springing up around the world. Database software has become increasingly user-friendly. Research libraries and even moderately sized community libraries buy site licenses to various indexes, and offer their clients free searching of CD-ROMs and mainframe-mounted indexes. The Internet offers direct access to both new and old sources of information.

The upshot of this revolution is that you need to know how to conduct a literature search yourself. Whether you consider this a blessing or a curse depends on your approach to the task and your knowledge of available resources.

23

Understand the strengths of different communication channels

The way scientists transmit their work to one another has changed more in the past two decades than it did in the preceding three centuries, dating back to the late seventeenth century when scholarly journals first appeared. Many new communication channels have opened, each differing in the kinds of information they transfer and in the restrictions that govern the ways information enters and exits.

Primary scientific communication can be thought of as informal or formal (Table 2.1). In addition, there are secondary channels that compile and evaluate materials obtained from the primary sources. No one branch is more or less important than another, but they operate in different ways. This makes it important that all of them be included in any comprehensive search for relevant information on a topic (Cooper, 1998).

Informal channels directly link researchers and literature sources

Informal communication channels include personal contact, personal solicitation, the traditional "invisible college" (and its cousin, the electronic invisible college or computer mailing list), and the World Wide Web. Informal communication is often one-on-one, occurring in person or through the mail, by telephone, and by exchange of reprints. Few explicit rules govern the contact between the scientist who has done the research and the person who is seeking to learn about its existence. There are few restrictions on the kinds of information that can be exchanged, and no third party mediates that exchange.

Personal contacts include all sorts of invaluable exchange. Students and professors share ideas back and forth. A colleague down the hall passes along an article he feels would be of interest. A reviewer notes a relevant paper that the author has missed. However, personal contact is generally a very restricted communication channel, for it depends on people who know each other and initiate the exchange.

Personal solicitation opens the channel a bit wider, and thus can produce less biased samples of information. After identifying groups of individuals who might have access to relevant research reports, a searcher would obtain lists and contact group members individually by telephone, mail, or email, to ask for relevant leads.

The term "invisible college" refers to informal but systematic ways that scientists arrange to stay in contact with colleagues who are working on similar problems. In the past, the lines of communication occurred primarily one-on-one, but with the advent of the Internet, they now are also maintained through computerized mailing list management programs and through newsgroups. Anyone can join mailing lists or newsgroups by sending a simple command to their host computer. Lists can be found in printed directories, in Internet directories, or by sending email instructions to "lists of lists" such as `<listserv@listserv.net>`. They can also be found by visiting Internet websites of research organizations.

Table 2.1. *Information pathways in a computer-aided literature system*

The flow of information	Formal communication channels	Informal communication channels
How information enters the system	Third party mediates the information that is exchanged	Information is directly exchanged
Examples of ways in which information enters the system	– refereed journals – invited talks at meetings – indexing services	– networking – refereeing – mailing lists – reprint exchanges – web pages

Examples of ways in which information is retrieved	– searching databases
	– surveying journals
	– examining article
	  references
	– attending talks at
	  meetings
		– getting email
		– receiving reprints
		– searching the Web

Output	User publishes bibliography or references section, making the information available by formal and informal pathways, and thus completing the cycle of information transfer	

The World Wide Web is a system of links between computers. Computer programs (servers) that provide a resource are linked to computer programs (clients) that wish to access that resource. The actual information exchanged is typically in the form of websites or webpages. These can be constructed by anyone who has (or knows someone who has) the required expertise. There is little restriction on whose information can enter the system. The problems of finding appropriate sites and evaluating them are discussed later in this chapter.

Formal channels involve third parties

The four major formal channels of scientific communication are professional conference presentations, personal journal libraries, electronic journals, and research report reference lists. If literature searching were courtship, informal channels would be face-to-face dates, but these formal channels would be blind dates arranged by friends. Formal channels of communication insert an element of judgment into the system. To enter information into them, researchers must follow explicit rules that restrict the kind or quality of information that is admitted into the system.

The traditional link between the primary researcher and the research synthesist is a classic example of a formal communication channel – an article published in a refereed scientific journal must follow specific requirements, and both editors and reviewers judge its acceptability. Research has shown that this review process also restricts information by tending to favor researchers whose work confirms currently held beliefs (Cooper, 1998).

Although their selection criteria for presentations is sometimes less strict than that required for journal publication, the conferences periodically held by various professional societies accept only presentations structured to their topic area. For information to enter the system, the researcher must be aware of the meeting, and the research generally must pass at least a weak peer review.

Relative to traditional journals, articles in electronic journals have much shorter publication lag times. Electronic journals use computer storage media such as Internet computer servers or CD-ROM to disseminate and archive full-text reports of scholarly work. Currently, some journals appear in both paper and electronic forms. However, due to the storage capacity and favorable economics of computer technology, many experts predict a gradual switch to solely electronic editions (Peek and Newby, 1996; Walker, 1998).

It is important to know which electronic journals do and do not evaluate submitted articles. A virtual library of electronic journals can be found at <http://gort.ucsd.edu/newjour/>. Clicking on any specific title sends the searcher to the electronic journal's homepage.

Compilations are there to help – use them!

Research bibliographies, research registers, reference databases, and citation indexes are compilations constructed for the explicit purpose of providing relatively comprehensive lists of published information related to a topic. They can be some of your most valuable literature searching sources.

Each of these databases has limitations, however. Some contain only published research and others only unpublished research. As with the Internet, one enters the database by specifying keywords; any mismatch between the seeker and the indexer is likely to result in missed articles. There can be a long time lag before references appear in an electronic index, because the study must be written, submitted, and published, then identified and catalogued into the reference database. It is not uncommon for a database to be a year or more behind. Physical browsing for newly appearing information is still advisable. Furthermore, despite their claims, none of the online databases include all the relevant journals on a topic. Use multiple sources.

Consult research bibliographies and research registers

Research bibliographies can be a great help and time-saver. They generally take the form of nonevaluative listings of books and articles relevant to a particular topic area, but it is even possible to find bibliographies of bibliographies. Research bibliographies are often maintained by single scientists or groups of individuals, rather than by a formal organization.

Prevalent in the medical sciences, research registers are databases of studies focusing on a common feature, such as subject matter, funding source, or design. Prospective research registers are unique in attempting to include not only completed research, but also research that is in the planning stage or is still under way. Some research registers are more comprehensive than others; whenever possible, determine how long a register has been in existence and how the research included in the register got to be there.

Locate and use reference databases and abstracting services

Reference databases (Table 2.2) are particularly fruitful sources of information. Maintained by both private and public organizations, these services focus on a specific kind of document (such as theses and dissertations) or field (such as agriculture or medicine). At present, most include only titles and abstracts, but full-text databases are becoming more prevalent and probably will be the norm in the future.

All major research libraries have reference databases, with reference librarians to help first-time users. Many databases are available in more than one medium. The older media (print, microfilm, microfiche and more recently CD-ROMs) require physically visiting the library.

Using online reference databases can save considerable time and ensure a high degree of accuracy. Furthermore, online reference databases are sometimes updated more frequently than their CD-ROM equivalents. Some databases are only available through licensed sites, such as a university library. Others can be accessed online through one's home or office computer, either by dialing up the commercial services or by using appropriate software to access them through the Internet.

Individual vendors and reference database publishers provide detailed and readily available instructions on database searching. Several excellent books are available as well, including *Library Use: A Handbook for Psychology*, prepared under the auspices of the American Psychological Association (Reed and Baxter, 1992) and *Coyle's Information Highway Handbook* (Coyle, 1997). Learn the shortcuts that make can make your life easier. For example, database software usually has the capacity to format references in a variety of ways, representative of the formats most commonly found in the scientific literature. Select the most up-to-date and versatile tools available, and take the time to master them.

Consult citation indexes and Dissertation Abstracts

Citation indexes are a unique kind of reference database that identifies and groups together all newly published articles that have referenced (cited) the same earlier publication. Citation indexes limit entries to references in published research, both journals and books, but are quite exhaustive within these categories.

Academia houses a great deal of potentially valuable but largely unpublished material in the form of doctoral dissertations and masters' theses. Although many reference databases contain abstracts of dissertations, *Dissertation*

Table 2.2. *Examples of helpful abstracting and indexing databases available to biological and medical researchers*

Database	Description
Agricola	Covers all major areas of agricultural sciences.
Agricultural and Environmental Biotechnology Abstracts	Especially useful for genetic engineering and its agricultural implications.
Bioengineering Abstracts	Covers biomedical and genetic engineering and related fields.
BIOSIS (Biological Abstracts)	Widely used for literature in biology, agriculture, and biomedicine. Includes five different indexes – author, genus, biosystematic grouping from phylum through family, concept, and subject. Records prior to 1993 are formatted and indexed differently from records since that time.
Biological and Agricultural Index	Particularly useful for environmental and conservation sciences, agriculture, veterinary medicine, and related areas of applied biology. Includes many periodicals devoted entirely to reviews.
Books in Print	Covers in-print, out-of-print, and forthcoming books from North American publishers.
CAB Abstracts	Excellent coverage for agriculture, veterinary medicine, and biology.
Cambridge Scientific Abstracts	The Biological Sciences Set and the Biotechnology and Engineering Set are particularly useful.
CINAHL (Cumulative Index to Nursing and Allied Health)	Particularly strong coverage of the nursing and allied health professions literature.
Current Contents	Indexes recent articles in a variety of life sciences by reproducing the tables of contents of numerous journals. Authors' addresses enable contact to request a copy of the paper if the journal is unavailable. Includes abstracts.
Dissertation Abstracts	Provides complete abstracts of dissertations from the U.S., Canada, Britain, and other countries, plus select coverage of masters theses.
General Science Index	Helpful place to start when working with a broad topic. Includes both papers in selected technical journals and nontechnical overviews, many of which are written by scientists who have also published technical papers on the same topic. (Locate the latter by searching by author names in more specialized daatabases.)

Table 2.2. *(cont.)*

Database	Description
Journal Citation Reports (an annual volume of *Science Citation Index*)	Lists indexed journals grouped by subject field. Ranks journals by their relative "impact factors," including number of citations of a journal's papers in other publications during a given calendar year and other statistics.
Medical and Pharmaceutical Biotechnology Abstracts	Covers human health, molecular biology, and biotechnology.
MEDLINE	The online counterpart to *Index Medicus*, and one of a group of databases (MEDLARS = Medical Literature Analysis and Retrieval System) produced by the U.S. National Library of Medicine. Includes all the medical and health sciences; unsurpassed for preclinical and clinical medicine.
Science Citation Index	Widely used to locate other authors who have mentioned a paper relevant to one's topic. Accompanying related indexes include the *Source Index*, with full bibliographic information on those papers; *Corporate Index*, which lists all articles originating at the same institution; and *Permuterm Subject Index*, which lists pairs of key terms, with titles that include both words in the pair.
Web of Science	Incorporates various searchable databases (including *Science Citation Index*) from the Institute of Scientific Information (ISI).
Zoological Record	The most comprehensive index to zoological literature.

Abstracts International focuses exclusively on them. Both the printed and the computerized versions include records dating back to 1861. The computerized version also includes abstracts of masters' theses back to 1962.

Obtaining the full text of theses and dissertations that are not physically housed nearby can be a nuisance. When an abstract appears relevant, you usually must use interlibrary loan to borrow a copy from the university at which the dissertation research was conducted. Alternatively, you may need to purchase a copy from University Microfilms International (UMI; Ann Arbor, Michigan); universities that maintain agreements with UMI are not allowed to lend dissertations through interlibrary loan.

Learn to use keyword search terms and apply Boolean logic

Most literature retrieval services are really matchmakers (Table 2.3). They have some provision for searching a subject by way of keywords – brief terms chosen (usually chosen by a study's author) to describe the major topics included in the

Table 2.3. *Using keywords and search logic to find a topic via computer-assisted searching*

What you enter	What sources are listed
Keywords (descriptors) that describe what you are looking for	Every source that contains those words in its title, text, or abstract.
Boolean terms	All sources that include: AND – both keywords OR – either keyword NOT – one keyword but not another.
Wildcard characters	All sources that contain the letters in the keyword plus any character or string of characters that appears in place of the wildcard asterisk.
Truncated descriptors	All sources that include the specified word root.
Proximity operators	All sources in which the keywords are within a certain number of words of each other.
A direct question	With search engines that support it, either sources to research, or a choice of questions that the software matches as being similar to the one you asked.

document. To find the document, one must specify the same keyword that the author has chosen (or a part of it; see wildcard characters).

Language gets much of its meaning through context, however. As a result, typing in keywords during an Internet search without specifying their context or relationships can lead to strange, frustrating, or humorous results. To improve the outcome, use a special system called Boolean logic to specify the relationships between search terms.

Boolean logic is named for George Boole, a mathematician who lived in the middle 1800s. It really is just a highbrowed way of describing three logical choices:

> I want this one AND that one
> I want this one OR that one
> I want this one but NOT that one

Search tools let you apply Boolean logic in various ways. With the system called Full Boolean, you type in AND, OR, and NOT (or in some systems, AND NOT) in capital letters to describe your choices. Suppose you wish to do a comparative study of types of skin cancer. By specifying carcinoma AND melanoma, you would retrieve all hits (entries computer-matched to your search) in which both types of cancers appear in the same document, but none that mention only one. For a comprehensive search on both kinds of skin cancer, you would specify carcinoma OR melanoma. Either or both terms would appear in each document that is retrieved. Alternatively, perhaps you want more information on skin cancers, but know that because of its potential deadliness, there will be hundreds of entries on malignant melanoma. To narrow the results, you could specify `carcinoma NOT melanoma`. Any document about skin cancer that mentioned melanoma would be omitted from the list of retrievals.

With the system called Implied Boolean, you use "logical operators," i.e., a plus sign in place of `AND` and a minus sign in place of `NOT`. The signs abut the front of the word, with no space between them. Precede this with other search terms you want to have it coupled with. For example, type `plastic facial +surgery` to get results for facial surgery and plastic surgery but not for the words plastic or facial alone. Use a minus sign in front of a word to ensure that a word does not appear in hits. For example, `poisoning -food` would yield information on poisoning without including entries on food poisoning.

Another variation allows you to choose from a menu of options that describe the Boolean logic, such as "all of these words," "any of these words," and "must not contain."

Plan an effective search strategy

For efficient use of time and energy, carefully define the scope of your literature review right at the beginning. How extensive do you want it to be? Do you want to get a broad list that includes records even slightly related to your topic, or just a few most relevant ones? To what extent do you need to rely upon informal channels versus formal ones?

Then, be prepared for a bit of trial-and-error. Identify a limited number of concepts that may be useful to describe the research question at hand, and choose terms and accompanying logic that seem to define them. Precision is imperative. Searching for instances of a broad term like `ecology` or `drugs` would be akin to drinking from a fire hose, summoning thousands of hits. The list that is returned often will display the total number of items found, but only show them in batches.

Run a computerized search using your initial set of terms, and look over a sample of the records it retrieves. Are they mostly relevant? If not, revise your search. To increase the number of records, expand the lists of terms connected by `OR`. To retrieve fewer records, narrow the search by adding terms or concepts connected by `AND` or (very carefully) by `NOT` logic. Most databases will let you define a time period or subject area for your search; many Internet searches still will not. Another useful capability of some online databases is the option of using an index tree or thesaurus. The vocabulary is arranged hierarchically, allowing the searcher to scroll through the list and select topics to broaden or narrow search parameters as desired.

When you are satisfied with the records obtained from one information channel, but feel you do not have everything that you need or want, begin all over again with another. The results will probably be different.

Handle search results wisely

Scientific papers nearly always conclude with a list of references or literature cited. Database software programs today are incredibly sophisticated and can

Exercise 2–1. Search strategy and Boolean logic

This is an exercise in thinking logically, not in finding answers on the Web. Here are ten publication titles. Use them to answer the questions below.

A. Trap-Nesting Wasps And Bees: Life Histories, Nests, And Associates
B. Behavior Of Three Florida Solitary Wasps
C. Winged Warriers: Insects In The Garden
D. A Cluster Of Bees
E. The Wasps Of The Genus *Pisonopsis* Fox
F. Beeswax, Twine and Time: The Art of Candlemaking
G. Cowfly Tigers: An Account Of The Bembicine Wasps Of British Guyana
H. Honeybees Attacked At Their Hive Entrance By *Philanthus* Wasps
I. A Life History of Stinging Insects
J. Comparative Study Of The Nesting Habits Of Solitary Bees And Wasps

Write the number(s) corresponding to the title(s) that would be retrieved for each of the following Boolean statements.

1. Wasps AND Bees   2. Wasps NOT Bees
3. Bees NOT Wasps   4. Wasps OR Bees

5. When using terms in a subject directory, you will usually get only relevant titles. When using terms in a search engine, you should expect a mixture of relevant and irrelevant titles. If you were searching for Wasps OR Bees using a search engine, which of the above titles would probably be retrieved but have little to do with them?

6. When you search one of the better subject directories, you search not only titles but annotations written by a staff person. Which of the above titles would be missed by a search engine using the keywords wasp OR bee, but might contain relevant information that would be retrieved by a good subject directory?

automatically format literature citations in any of the most widely used journal formats. They can be integrated with word processor programs to format the references within a typescript and allow introduction of references during typescript preparation.

Nevertheless, you must exercise care and vigilance when entering reference citations into your personal database. While it can be tempting to add bibliographic references to your personal database from the literature cited sections of review articles and other publications, avoid doing so. It is a good idea to devise a system to indicate whether you have personally verified the correctness of a bibliographic entry. Never trust the accuracy of others (Blanchard, 1974). A useful operating procedure is to never incorporate a reference into your database unless you have actually verified it.

USE THE INTERNET WISELY AND WELL

As a successful writer, you will find yourself using the Internet repeatedly. This vast, interconnected system of smaller public and private networks lets users communicate around the globe, finding and sharing information, offering commercial services, and opening vast information resources.

A popular analogy likens the Internet to a library, but if so the Internet is a strange library indeed. Titles may not be terribly descriptive and exact authors are often unclear. What it calls a page does not correspond with standard paper sizes or a computer screen. What it calls a site isn't a place at all. If you know a site's electronic label (URL), finding it is easy; the name includes its "shelf location." However, if you don't, it can be difficult or even impossible to find. The partial catalogs that are available each classify content in different ways and because there is no complete listing anywhere, you have no way of knowing whether you have found everything that is there. Furthermore, as a relatively new resource, the Internet is an ever-changing entity. Printed material pointing to specific sites is sometimes outdated before it is even published. Finding something useful once doesn't mean you will be able to locate it again.

The secret to dealing with this vast, chaotically organized resource and its instability is learning to understand how it works and how to use specialized tools designed to facilitate your scientific writing efforts.

Know how the Internet is structured

The Internet is a global network of computers, linked by a common language (TCP/IP); the revolutionary aspect of this language is simply that it allows communication between computers using diverse operating systems that could not previously share information. Many methods of communicating between these linked computers have been developed (Table 2.4), spawning a whole new interactive environment that is fundamentally different from passive media such as television or print. (It also has given rise to a whole set of jargon; see Table 7.3 on page 145.)

Although many people erroneously equate them, the World Wide Web is not the Internet, but only one of many services, each with slightly different strengths, weaknesses, and operating procedures. Any computer with an Internet connection and the necessary software can use any of them, and the same server often offers several choices. Sometimes the Web is the best place to search for information; in other cases, another choice might be more appropriate.

Table 2.4. *Some basic types of Internet resources of interest to scientists*

Type of resource	Purpose	Nonelectronic equivalent	How to access the resource from a computer with modem and Internet connection
LISTSERV	To find and communicate with people who share interests	Round-robin letters or being on a mailing list	Message automatically arrives with email; many listservs also have archives of past messages.
Usenet (newsgroups)	To access a global collection of interest groups that share news	A specialty newsletter to read at your convenience	Use a newsreader (software that allows you to access and manage discussion group messages).
email (electronic mail)	To correspond with one or more people directly	Letters sent back and forth between individuals or groups	Use an email program or choose one of the free web-based email services.
World Wide Web (WWW, or Web)	An umbrella application that supports all the above, plus information organized into "pages" identified by unique URL addresses	A worldwide library with audiovisual and communication facilities	Use a client program called a "browser" to search for a URL from any computer with an Internet connection.
Gopher	To find information organized using hierarchical menu structures	The same library, with its contents more systematically organized	Navigate up and down menus with Gopher client software or use a Web browser.
File Transfer Protocol (FTP)	To move files around the Internet, downloading software applications and other files to your personal computer and/or uploading from the PC to a server	A television game show with prizes	Some FTP sites require passwords, but most do not. Some downloaded files may need to be converted into a readable format.

Table 2.4. *(cont.)*

Type of resource	Purpose	Nonelectronic equivalent	How to access the resource from a computer with modem and Internet connection
Telnet	To connect to other computers on the Internet and use those computers and their software applications as though you were physically present	Science-fiction teleporting	Most telnet sites require a password, a user name, or other log-in language. In addition to telnet client software, you can use a Web browser to access sites.

One might imagine the Internet as a supermarket, with the Web as a large and enticing produce section (Hoffman, 1995). It might be the only section you visit if you are looking for carrots, but you might bypass it entirely if you were dropping in to pick up a loaf of bread. Furthermore, while the produce section contains primarily fresh fruits and vegetables, sometimes one also finds miscellaneous nonproduce items such as salad dressing there, and bananas may appear again over in the cereal aisle.

Understand Web addresses

To access a site (domain) on the Internet, you need its unique address, which is called its URL (Uniform Resource Locator). To access a particular website, simply type in the URL exactly as it appears, without any extra spaces. Note that any punctuation that appears in the URL is also an essential part of the address. For example, a biology curriculum development project has the full address:

```
<http://entomology.ent.uga.edu/wowbugs/index.html>
```

Although it may look like gibberish at first glance, each part has a specific meaning. Separated by punctuation, they include the protocol, domain, directory path, and page name. The protocol describes how the information is to be transferred, i.e., which Internet service is being accessed. The most common protocol is http, and many web browsers fill this in automatically when you type in the rest of the URL. Other common protocols include ftp (file transfer protocol), gopher, mailto, and news.

The domain name consists of two or more parts separated by single dots. It often begins with www, and many web browsers now also fill this in automatically. The first or central part of the domain consists of a code for the name of the organization (and sometimes the specific computer at the organization). In the example above, it is the Entomology Department's server at the University of Georgia.

The last part is called the top-level domain. In the United States, it tells you the type of organization that is hosting the site. These include:

.com	for commercial entities
.edu	for educational institutions (usually universities)
.gov	for governmental entities
.mil	for the military services
.net	for a company providing networking services
.org	for nonprofit organizations

In late 1996, a proposal was made to add seven new top-level domains to keep up with the growth of the Internet. Thus, you may also see:

.arts	for entities emphasizing culture and entertainment
.firm	for businesses and firms
.info	for entities providing information services
.nom	for those wishing individual or personal nomenclature
.rec	for entities emphasizing recreational entertainment and activities
.store	for businesses offering goods to purchase
.web	for entities emphasizing activities related to the Web

Top-level domain names often also identify a country of origin (such as ca for Canada, or ch for Switzerland). A complete list of country codes can be found at:

<http://metalab.unc.edu/pub/docs/rfc/rfc1394.txt>

Every URL has at least a protocol and domain; many also include the full path through a directory or folder to a specific file. The final URL entries are directions to the machine that hosts the Web pages you are seeking. First comes a portion (such as wowbugs/) that specifies a directory within the machine's file structure. In the wowbugs example there is only one level, but larger websites may have numerous subdirectories. This is followed by the name of the specific file you are requesting. The entry named index.html indicates that no specific file is requested.

Know what Gopher is

For academic researchers, Gopher is a popular system to retrieve data from universities, companies, and other organizations. Gopher became popular around the same time that the Web was invented, and at first it was the more popular Internet service. Its protocol is simpler, but it lacks formatted text, so it looks more primitive and less interesting. However, its onscreen appearance is also more predictable, and the information is neatly organized. Web-based search tools can be used to conduct searches of Gopher sites; there are also specialized search tools for them.

Appreciate FTP

With FTP (anonymous file transfer protocol), all you see are directory names and file names. But although it looks old-fashioned, FTP is a remarkably resilient system still used by all the major file repositories and many file duplication utilities. It provides a way to retrieve (and copy, at no cost) a huge and ever expanding number of public files from host computers all over the Internet. This "public access" material includes documents, audio and video clips, and even software that can be downloaded to your computer.

Archie is the name of the preferred searching system for files in anonymous FTP archives. Archie servers throughout the world enable you to log in or use Archie client software to search for files and directories by their titles. Note, however, that many server sites have both an FTP server and a Gopher or Web server viewing the same files. The Web server software can add formatting that makes the directories a bit more informative, and spares you the character-based FTP client software and its myriad of arcane commands.

Be aware of telnet

Telnet was one of the very first Internet services to be developed, but today it is used primarily to access University library catalogs, computer bulletin board systems, and sometimes email. Few Web clients offer built-in support for it. Instead, they start a different program, which you must have on your computer to run the telnet session. Consequently, many people never use telnet.

When you telnet to another computer, it has the same effect as using a modem to dial up the other computer. However, once you reach the other computer, there is no easy way to determine how to interact with it. Libraries use dozens of different systems to access their catalogs, making it difficult to figure out what commands will give you access.

Learn the differences between subject directories and search engines

What if you don't know what information is out there, or where it is located? There are two different approaches to searching for information on the World Wide Web (Table 2.5). One is the subject directory approach. Browse or search a small database of titles and annotations that people have preselected and organized into subject categories. The other is the search engine approach. Search an enormous database that includes the full text of each resource but is not organized into categories.

Note, however, that like everything else in the online universe, the clearcut division between subject directories and search engines is changing. Some searching tools such as Magellan Internet Guide at <www.mckinley.com> already include both a search engine and a subject directory.

Table 2.5. *Examples of major Internet search tools (URLs subject to change)*

Subject directories	Search engines
Yahoo!	AltaVista
`www.yahoo.com`	`www.altavista.com`
The Argus ClearingHouse	Hotbot
`www.clearinghouse.net`	`hotbot.lycos.com`
WebCrawler	Infoseek
`www.webcrawler.com`	`infoseek.go.com`
Librarians' Index to the Internet	Lycos
`sunsite.berkeley.edu/`	`www.lycos.com`
`InternetIndex`	
Scholarly Internet Resource Collection	Excite
`infomine.ucr.edu`	`www.excite.com`
	Northern Light
	`www.northernlight.com`

Use broad and inclusive terms to search subject directories

Subject directories are specialized websites that select other sites and organize them under broad subject headings to browse through or search by keywords. No two directories categorize their materials in the same way, and each directory covers only a small subset of the entire Internet. Yahoo!, the largest and most popular subject directory, covers less than 5% of the Web (Gould, 1998). The strength of subject directories lies in the human touch; resources are categorized by general topic, not specific vocabulary.

To use subject directories most effectively, choose broad, inclusive keywords because unique terms will often yield no results. Keep in mind, however, that failure to find information does not mean it does not exist. The directory simply may not have picked it up for indexing.

Prefer narrowly defined and unusual terms with search engines

Unlike subject directories, search engines are software programs that consist of comprehensive indexes of the Internet. You can find a catalog of them, listed by category, at <`search.cnet.com`>. Their (nearly impossible) goal is to index every word of every Web page in their databases, but even the biggest search engines index only 60–80% of the Web (Gould, 1998). Their databases are created by computer programs – variously called robots, spiders, or web-crawlers – that work constantly to collect and index Web pages.

To query a search engine, you must provide keyword clues to what you are seeking (refer back to Table 2.3). The computer will attempt to honor your request with a ranked list ("hit" list) of sites. However, because so much information is available, it is common to get overloaded with results that mix trivial or irrelevant results with the pertinent ones. Search engines attempt to help with this problem by applying ranking algorithms or formulas that determine the order in which the results are displayed. Small differences in these algorithms have a major effect on the results obtained, even when you use identical search terms. Get in the habit of never relying on results from only one search engine.

To use search engines effectively, choose very specific keywords and combine them in an appropriate syntax to take advantage of advanced search features. The more uncommon the word or phrase, the more manageable the number of retrievals will be, and the fewer irrelevant documents that will appear. Avoid keywords such as `Internet`, `and`, `of`, or `help`, which are so common that many search engines ignore them completely.

Take advantage of advanced search features

As the Web continues to grow, or as your research needs dictate, you will probably find it increasingly important to use special features that allow you to refine and focus your searches more precisely. For example, many search engines allow you to use quotation marks to surround words that you want to have kept together in their specified order. This enables searches for entire phrases rather than individual words. Thus you would type ``paper wasp'' when you want information on the insect. Without the quotes, you would also retrieve documents about places to buy paper, how to make paper at home, and information about all kinds of wasps, not just paper wasps.

Because computerized searches rely on a simple matching process, the essential core of a word is enough to find its many variations. At its simplest, this means singular keywords will also identify the plural of those words, but not vice versa. Searching for `tubule` will find `tubules`, but searching for `tubules` will not recognize a title that says only `tubule`.

Truncation and wildcard characters are two allied features to use when you aren't sure of a correct spelling or you want to retrieve many forms of a word. Symbols vary with the program, but the asterisk (*) is the most commonly used wildcard character. It can be used in place of one or more letters in a keyword, such as searching `amar*is` when you are not sure of the spelling for the amaryllis flower, or `arch*ology` for the twin spellings of archaeology and archeology.

Stemming is the name of the related process of stripping a term of suffixes to find its "root" to use as a truncated search term. Some search tools stem automatically. There are also specialized dictionaries of word roots to help find all possible word variants of a term. When done automatically or carelessly, however, stemming and truncation often result in too many irrelevant hits and become more hindrance than help.

Proximity operators allow you to specify where terms appear relative to one another. With NEAR they must be within a certain number of words of each other. With FOLLOWED BY, just as with a phrase search, the first term must be followed by the second. With ADJACENT the words must be next to one another, but can appear in either order. The entry Voyage AND Beagle NEAR Darwin should find "Darwin's Voyage of the Beagle" or "when Darwin took his famous voyage on the Beagle" without also retrieving irrelevant entries on dogs or lunar voyages.

Keep your eyes and mind open to new services

In an attempt to differentiate themselves from the competition, search sites offer an increasing variety of search services. For example, some websites provide "one-stop-shopping" search services called metasearch engines. One of the oldest examples is found at <www.allonesearch.com>. In addition to making it easier to conduct a search without having to go to each search tool individually, such sites are useful because they give you easy access to search sites that you may be unaware of or may have forgotten.

What about other Internet services? Dozens of them are not yet represented on the Web. However, nothing prevents them from being there, and some may have arrived by the time you read this. Many are already available through a website called a gateway. This is a program that translates between two protocols; it operates somewhat like an automated dictionary for two human languages (Hoffman, 1995).

Keep the Internet in perspective

Unlike most library-based research material, much information on the Internet in general and the World Wide Web in particular is still largely the work of enthusiastic amateurs. You must be the judge of how accurate and useful materials are, for these resources include a jumble of advertisements, one-sided statements, and false information mixed in with good, reliable data. Rely on the same kind of critical thinking you use to assess the usefulness of a print source. For an excellent discussion with practical suggestions on this topic, read *Digital Literacy* (Gilster, 1997).

The Internet and especially the World Wide Web are undeniably new and exciting. However, there is a common misconception that with their arrival, literature searching has become a breeze. Reality is closer to a description by Gould (1998, p. 8):

If you keep in mind that the Internet just came out of the trees and got into the knuckle-walking stage of its evolution, you will be able to appreciate what is there, and reduce your frustration at working in this very young medium.

USE EMAIL AS A TIME-SAVING RESOURCE

Electronic communication via email is now commonplace. Within minutes of being written, messages are received even at vast distances from the sender. Here they reside in a computer file called an electronic mail box, until the recipient wants to display and read them on the screen, print them as a permanent record, forward them to others, save them to a disk or hard drive, or reply to the original sender.

As a successful scientific writer, you will be using email often. Because emailed information is transmitted in machine-readable form, the text can be printed, revised, and sent back, or even incorporated directly into another computer file without being retyped. These abilities can be used to your advantage in many ways. References, abstracts, and even entire articles located in a particular database can be directed to your personal email address. There you can download them, then print a copy or add them directly to your computerized literature retrieval system.

With the ability to send even lengthy documents as attachments to email messages, collaborative typescript preparation has never been easier. You can correspond rapidly with colleagues around the globe, seek and give advice and suggestions, and work together more closely than has ever been possible. Even when you work on collaborative writing projects with the person across the hall, you can send drafts back and forth between team members for comment, and receive and incorporate those comments electronically.

To use email wisely and well, however, heed a few points of online etiquette.

Pay attention to details in email addresses

Many email addresses are very similar. To be sure your messages end up where you want them to, address them carefully. If you use a preset address list, click carefully. Stories abound regarding people who sent a message to the wrong person, with disastrous or humorous results.

Follow the capitalization exactly in address lines. Many systems are case sensitive. Some companies use capitals in the middle of their own or their products' name, effectively turning two words into one. Follow the style you see in their advertising or on the product itself.

Watch out for unintended consequences if you address an email message to a long list of people, either as primary recipients or through carbon copies. Some programs cannot handle more than a limited number of addresses, and will cut off the additional ones. Others will string the text across more and more of the page in an attempt to make it match. If you are uncertain how your program is handling these, send a trial message to some friends and ask for their comments.

Be civil, circumspect, and courteous

While email has transformed communication between colleagues, a few cautions are in order. Email messages tend to be less formal and more conversational than most science-related writing, both because of the immediacy of the transmission and because it usually occurs directly between two people. Avoid writing poorly, inaccurately, or inadvisably. Whether during a quick one-on-one reply to a colleague or within the seeming anonymity of forums such as chat rooms, never be tempted to dash off strongly worded or ill-advised statements. Remember, verbal harassment or other inconsiderate language, called flaming, is as ill-advised online as it is in face-to-face encounters.

Writing or reading email may seem like a solitary activity, but in fact email messages are much like the old party line telephones. They can be read or printed by someone other than the intended recipient, not only during transmission but subsequent to it. Consider all your messages in the light of this possibility.

Make your messages easy to read

Reading email text on a computer screen can be difficult. Make it as easy for your recipient as you can. Use normal punctuation. Words all in capital letters, which look like shouting, will annoy your recipients. All lowercase also is annoying, because it is hard to read and looks as though you don't care enough to punctuate.

With no font diversity, italics, or boldfacing to offer variety, long chunks of online text are especially difficult to read on the screen. If your program does not allow paragraph indenting, break text into short block paragraphs, leaving some extra space between each one.

Substitute for italics, if necessary

Italic type is an integral part of most scientific writing, but some online communication programs do not allow its use. In a manuscript, one would underline words instead, but on the World Wide Web underlining often signals an active hypertext link. Therefore, the usual convention is to substitute asterisks when italics would add emphasis to a word or phrase:

> The following precautions *must* be followed when doing this experiment.

To indicate a title or a scientific name, a common convention is to use the underline mark immediately before and after the otherwise-italicized material. Some writers use <bital> for begin italics and <eital> for end italics.

> That information appears in _Successful Scientific Writing_.

> Unlike _Melittobia_, the genus_Arpactophilus_ builds silk-lined nests.

> Matthews, R. W. 1996. Weird wonderful WOWBugs. <bital>Carolina Tips<eital> 60: 9-11.

FRANK & ERNEST® by Bob Thaves

FRANK AND ERNEST © NEA. Reprinted by permission.

USE WORD PROCESSING TO WRITE MORE EFFICIENTLY

The words come out of you like toothpaste sometimes.
Garrison Keillor

It is no longer news that a computer with appropriate software can function as a word processor, allowing even children to type, revise, and print text with minimal effort. By all means, use one to compose your scientific paper, right from the beginning. Insert and delete words or passages and rearrange text without repetitious retyping. With a single command, change a word or a spelling throughout the manuscript. From the first draft to the last, the word processor will save hours of time.

Even if a journal accepts only paper copy, using a word processor is worthwhile for an author. However, many journals are now accepting electronic submissions either as disk copy or through email. This is a welcome development for everyone involved, for it also saves money and decreases the probability of errors creeping into the final publication.

Use automatic formatting to save time and ensure consistency

When mastered, this feature can be used to set up a style for almost any purpose, from a letter, typescript, or journal article to an address list. Merrily type away and the computer will format the material, automatically handling such mundane details as paragraph indentation, hyphenation, pagination, and heading styles.

Automatic formatting can save considerable time when used on lengthy reference lists, in particular. An additional advantage of automatic formatting becomes evident if that format later must be modified. One simple change to the style sheet will update all occurrences of text formatted with a given style.

Nothing in a word-processed typescript need be numbered or alphabetized manually. Outline headings, paragraphs, columns in a table, and reference lists are but a few of the typescript components that can be sorted.

Numbered lists are particularly common in scientific writing, being used to present step-by-step instructions and outlines, and for other situations in which the specific order of information is important. Cultivate the time-saving habit of using automatic rather than manual numbering. When changes add material or rearrange its order, the program will automatically readjust so that items retain their sequential numbers.

Some journals require that lines of text be numbered in the left margin to allow editors to refer authors to specific passages. In the past, this required the use of special paper, and changes in text necessitated retyping the entire typescript. With the proper command, word-processing programs now will number lines automatically as the document is printed, either page by page or from the beginning of the typescript to its end.

Create tables without the hassle of setting tabs

Once upon a time, setting up tables was one of the most time-consuming parts of typescript preparation. Tabs were set, and column widths were adjusted by eye. The initial product looked fine, but later changes created havoc, scrambling column entries and making a general mess of the table.

Tables prepared by word processing look superficially like electronic spreadsheets, but commands set up expandable text entry areas (cells) that adjust to the size of the entries within them. Text is kept within these cells, where all manner of alterations can be made without affecting adjacent cells. Columns or rows can be added or subtracted at any time, and the table layout can be altered easily by adjusting column widths and changing row alignment. Recent versions of some popular word-processing software even allow for drag-and-drop alterations in the size and number of table elements.

Note that a frequently used table matrix can be stored as a glossary entry or shell. This can save considerable time when a lengthy typescript includes a number of similarly formatted tables.

Use special features to handle mathematics

For extensive computation, a spreadsheet program is still preferred. However, many useful calculations also can now be performed directly within word-processing programs. These include adding rows or columns of figures, multiplying or dividing numbers, and determining percentages. Calculations can be performed on numbers scattered throughout a document. Such features make it possible to build and edit numerical tables directly on the screen. Furthermore, results will be automatically updated if the figures in the table change, much as they are in a spreadsheet. Use these built-in capabilities to speed up the writing of reports, proposals, and other straightforward scientific documents.

Software for generating complex formulas is now widely available. As scientific journals increasingly turn to preparing issues directly from files submitted on disk, the ability to set up complex mathematical equations onscreen will become increasingly valuable. However, some journals may continue to prefer that complex mathematics be submitted as artwork or a glossy print. This can be accomplished easily, of course, with a laser-printed copy of the onscreen material.

Use hidden text for notes

This feature can speed the writing of a first draft because it allows the equivalent of secret parenthetical notes throughout the typescript. When characters are formatted as hidden text, they do not appear on the screen (or in print) without a specific command. They are equivalent to notes jotted in the margin. This feature is extremely useful in collaborative writing situations. Notes, annotations, or commentary can be inserted as desired by any author, and colleagues can call these up without affecting the typescript itself.

Because much of modern-day science is collaborative, coauthors each should have the opportunity to independently work on revising and improving the manuscript draft. Rather than circulating a single disk copy, it is more efficient and time saving for each to work on their own copy concurrently. Current word-processing programs allow for revisions to be inserted and clearly marked so that they can be easily spotted later and dealt with. It is also easy to "write-protect" a document with a password so that permanent changes cannot be made at this stage. Even so, always save a backup copy of the original draft before sharing it among collaborators.

Even though several individuals may independently suggest revisions to a manuscript, no longer is it necessary to manually transfer such changes from paper to computer. Most word-processing programs have the ability to merge hidden text annotations and revisions from different file copies of the manuscript onto a single master copy.

Hidden text also can be used for special commands that mark entries for a table of contents and index. This can be particularly useful when one wishes to index a concept rather than specific words. (An index also can be based directly on a search for the occurrences of specific words, a less powerful technique but one which is still faster than the old handwritten index-card method.)

Plan ahead to make revisions easier

No matter how many changes you make to the screen copy, plan to edit a printed typescript at some point. Never correct a document solely on the screen. Individuals tend to see different things when shuffling papers and making handwritten corrections than when scrolling through screen copy.

Whatever the eventual format of your typescript will be, plan to print out a copy with double-spaced lines and wide margins. An inch of margin on each side, with at least an inch on the top and bottom, is not excessive. Use a standard font in a reasonable size, such as 12-point Arial, Helvetica, Times New Roman, or New York.

Number pages automatically in a header or footer (a separate text block that contains information repeated at each page top or bottom, respectively). Include a brief identifying name for the typescript and (especially in collaborative writing situations) your own name. To visually distinguish the header or footer from the text, consider formatting this material in a different font and smaller point size and including extra space around it.

Command the program to insert a date and/or time into the header or footer, as well. These fields are particularly useful when more than one person is working on a document, or when a document goes through several revisions. Dates and times can either be frozen, or can reflect the current date and time each time a document is opened or printed.

Save your work often, and always make backups

Word processors do lose material – both during and after you've worked on it – and you must take extra steps to safeguard yourself from this catastrophe. When writing material out by hand, you can afford the luxury of plowing along nonstop for as long as the inspiration is with you. If you work this way with a word processor without saving material frequently, you're skating on thin ice.

During every working session, save your document at regular intervals. If a power failure or other problem causes the program to shut down while you are working, you can recover everything entered up until the last save command. If your program has the option of automatically saving documents, learn how to use this feature.

For extra security, keep a backup copy on disk in a separate location, or consider emailing the file as an attachment to a colleague or yourself. Remember, there are only two types of computer users – those who have lost files, and those who will.

REVISING WITH A WORD PROCESSOR

I now can quickly spell hors d'oeuvres
which grates on many people's nerves.
Unknown

The incredible capabilities of modern word-processing programs have ushered in an exciting new era, blurring the lines between writing and editing. They can have a profound psychological effect, for they ease one's transition back and forth from the role of writer to critical reader and back again. However, be somewhat wary and not too easily seduced by bells and whistles. Some new tools can distract one from the writing task at hand; others can be a tremendous productivity booster when mastered.

Use special features to revise material easily on the screen

For example, become familiar with the "search" or "find" feature. Not only can you find and change words or characters throughout the typescript with a single keystroke, you can also use these features to standardize format and to instantly locate and scroll to specific sections of the typescript.

This feature is often combined with a "replace" option, which can be very handy but needs to be used with care. For example, suppose you wished to replace the word "one" with "two" throughout your typescript. Since such a short word often happens to be part of another word, you would find all sorts of interesting but nonsensical words peppered throughout the text. Questioned would now be *questitwod*; telephone, *telephtwo*; done, *dtwo*. Avoid this predicament by specifying "whole words only." If your word processor has a thesaurus feature, use it to help make your prose more varied and interesting. Turn to it if you experience a mental block and can't come up with the right word. Try a possible synonym and let the thesaurus suggest and substitute alternative choices.

PEANUTS   by Charles Schulz

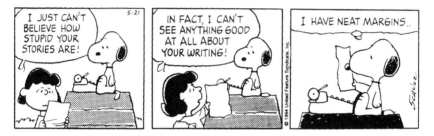

© United Feature Syndicate, Inc. Reprinted with permission.

Resist premature cosmetic work

Because it is so easy to make superficial changes, it is tempting to make each draft technically perfect, with every comma in place, every word spelled correctly, every margin perfectly aligned. Then, because the paper looks so good, one becomes rather hesitant to change it further, even though the basic structure may need a major overhaul. A paper like this can be compared to a beautifully painted house with termites – lovely outside but unsound within. Trust us – it's unlikely to fool editors and reviewers.

Furthermore, because the manuscript looks so good, many people find it difficult to throw away unnecessary material. If you find you've strayed off course, and ended up with more verbiage or material than you really need, cut out the extra, no matter how hard you worked at it. Some writers save their trimmings in a separate "orphan" file. Adopting a similar approach could be useful in case you change your mind later.

Use computerized grammar-checking programs wisely, if at all

Grammar-checking and style analysis programs are now widely available either as part of word-processing programs or as separate software. However, unlike a spellchecker, which is fairly mechanical and straightforward, a grammar checker requires a great deal of personal judgment. Each word, phrase, or passage that it questions must be considered individually to decide whether the program truly has flagged an error. In most cases, this is more time intensive than relying upon the grammar checker built into one's own neural anatomy.

Style analysis programs are most helpful for picking up simple mechanical problems, such as a missing parenthesis or quotation mark. Some will alert you to commonly misused words such as affect and effect. They will identify redundant, overworked, wordy, or trite phrases, and can help you detect noun-heavy passages by counting prepositions. They also can pick up writing quirks, such as too many short sentences or overuse of "to be" verbs. However, they flag only items that can be detected by pattern-matching. For this reason, errors such as subject–verb agreement – a particular problem in scientific writing – often slip by. Logic is completely beyond them, and they will approve a completely incomprehensible document if it appears in a form that passes for Standard Written English.

To date, style analysis programs are not very closely targeted to biomedical writing. They tend to flag a great many passages that do not need revision. For example, they may question every instance of the passive voice, even when used appropriately in scientific writing. Some packages allow you to disable the passive voice rule and certain other rules, but many idiosyncrasies inherent to the topic of your scientific paper will probably be questioned over and over again.

Writing experts stress that organization and coherence are the main determinants of writing quality. These are beyond the scope of any available editing program. Trying to use one of these programs while composing a first draft wastes time and promotes writer's block. The most efficient time to use a grammar-checking or style analysis program, if at all, is near the end of the writing process, after the document has been shuffled into a reasonable organization and polished to a reasonable degree of coherency, style, and grace. At this point, a grammar checker can provide one more way to ferret out undetected mechanical errors that might cause embarrassment.

Use a spellchecker but never entrust it with everything

The ability to check spelling is one of the strengths and blessings of word processing. Take advantage of it. More than that – make its use a regular habit. Professional writing requires perfect spelling. Misspelled words and typographical errors are viewed by many people as signs of carelessness, lack of professionalism, or limited intelligence – hardly the impression one wants to make on an editor or reviewer!

Run a spellchecker on every document that will leave your computer. It will speed your work, improve its accuracy, and spare you from becoming delayed by manual dictionary searches to check the spelling of seldom-used

---

Exercise 2–2. Grammar and style analysis programs

Enjoy these examples inspired by *Anguished English* (Lederer, 1987). Then rewrite the sentences to correct the errors a grammar checker would miss.

1. Migraines strike twice as many women as do men.

2. Wanted: Worker to take care of cow that does not smoke or drink.

3. As a baboon who grew up wild in the jungle, I realized that Wiki had special nutritional needs.

4. The patient was referred to a psychiatrist with a severe emotional problem.

5. In the photograph, veterinarian Joe Mobbs hoists a cow injured while giving birth to its feet.

6. About two years ago, a wart appeared on his left hand, which he wanted removed.

7. People who use birth control methods that smoke are in danger of having retarded children.

8. The woman wants to have the dog's tail operated on again, and if it doesn't heal this time, she'll have to be euthanized.

---

words. Most spellcheckers have several built-in dictionaries in various languages. In the United States, the main dictionary usually is called English Dictionary. However, there are many differences between American, Australian, and British spellings of English words. The customization feature will allow you to open one or more of these variant dictionaries, either singly or simultaneously.

Spellcheckers can be used for more than their name suggests. Faced with a word that is not in their dictionary, most spellcheckers will display a list of one or more potential choices. This feature can be a tremendous time-saver when one knows only approximately how to spell a word or when trying to think of a word one cannot quite remember. Make a best guess, and count on being able to recognize the word when it appears on the list.

At a command such as "change all," most spellcheckers will correct a word's spelling throughout the entire document without further need for confirmation. This feature can also be used like a "find and replace" command to change one word to an entirely different one.

Use a spellchecker to catch repeated words or errors in spacing. The best spellcheckers will do this automatically. This can be an important advantage, for

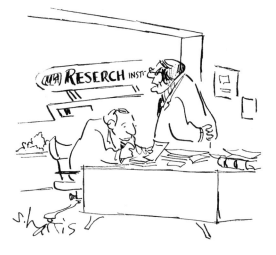

"GARFIELD, I THINK I KNOW WHY WE'VE
BEEN RECEIVING SO FEW COMMISSIONS."

Reprinted by permission of Sydney Harris.

repeated words (such as *this this*) and run-on words (such as *thisandthis*) are easy to overlook during proofreading.

At the same time, recognize a spellchecker's limitations. First, spellcheckers don't really check spelling. Instead, they compare the words in a document with correctly spelled words that are stored in the program's dictionaries. If the computer cannot find a match, it flags the word as unknown. Because it operates in this way, a spellchecker will not catch correctly spelled words used in the wrong context. A word can be correctly spelled and still be wrong – as in the case of homonyms, or the use of a correctly spelled word with the wrong meaning or tense. One cannot expect it to catch such errors as using *their* for *there*, nor can it catch misspellings that form other words. For example, omission of one letter changes *underserved* to *undeserved*, significantly changing the meaning. Nothing can substitute for a final human proofreading.

Second, a spellchecker is only as good as the words entered in its dictionary. Specialized terms, most names of people and places, and many commonly used scientific abbreviations and acronyms are generally absent. The words in the main dictionary of a spellchecker cannot be accessed; they are stored in a special, compressed file format. (Furthermore, if an incorrectly spelled word were added to this dictionary, the error could not be repaired.)

Building a user-accessible custom dictionary lessens the number of flagged words that appear. Because searching a custom dictionary takes longer than searching the main dictionary, savvy writers keep custom dictionaries short by building them by subject. One for general correspondence might include proper nouns such as street and city names; one for grant writing might contain

---

Exercise 2–3. Spellcheckers

Find the errors that the spellchecker missed in these sentences inspired by Lederer (1987).

1.   The young of the hoatzin, curious foul native to South America, are remarkable in having clawed fingers on their wings, by moans of which they are able to climb about trees like quadruplets.

2.   These imported trees are so profligate they are crowding out the more fragile naive species.

3.   The client has a congenial hip disease.

4.   He has been a prostrate patient for many years.

5.   The animals that normally inhabit the pond were dyeing because it had too much green allergy.

6.   The experimental group included three Great Dames and eight puppies from a German Shepherd and an Alaskan Hussy.

7.   She had a seizure, fell, and went unconscious. She was in a comma, and she never woke up.

8.   The pistol of a flower is it's only protection against insects.

9.   The doctor advised the patent to rest until the stitches were out and that there would be a permanent scare.

10. Our Spellwriter has the power to check wards within a document in as many as eight different languages, and this is only the tap of the iceberg.

---

common governmental acronyms and agencies; still another might contain the technical terms, Latin binomials, and proper nouns needed to spellcheck a research manuscript.

When you build a custom dictionary specifically for your scientific writing, be sure the words are spelled correctly when you enter them. Useful authoritative resources for specialized biomedical vocabulary include *Stedman's Medical Dictionary* (1995), *Dorland's Illustrated Medical Dictionary* (1994), *Handbook of Current Medical Abbreviations* (1998), and *Medical Terms and Abbreviations* (1998). See also Budavari (1998), Campbell and Campbell (1995), Holt *et al.* (1994), and Jablonski (1998). If you regularly write papers replete with specialized medical terminology, consider investing in medical dictionary software, which includes both definitions and specialized spellchecking.

Proofread the final version on paper

Spellcheckers assume that if a word is correctly spelled, it is the correct word. However, you may have chosen the wrong word. Thus, the last steps in manuscript revision should be your own careful proofreading of a paper copy, and a read-through by the most finicky person you know!

It is not easy to proofread your own material well. By the time you have worked through several drafts, you are no longer as observant as you might be. You will tend to read what you think is there, not what is actually on the page. One way around this is to pair up with someone else. As one of you reads aloud from one copy of the paper, the other should follow along on a written copy. If you must go it alone, it is best if you can lay the manuscript aside for a period of time before proofreading it. A fresh start makes it more likely that errors or stylistic flaws will be detected.

Guard your investment

Continue to save work frequently and make backups. The more time and energy you have invested in a document, the more important it is to protect that investment. A bit of paranoia can be healthy. Keep a duplicate copy on a second disk as a safeguard against inadvertently erasing the first file. Remember to update the backup file each time you make revisions. When you are not working on the computer, store the disks in different places.

3

Writing the first draft

Writing is easy. All you do is stare at a blank sheet of paper
until drops of blood form on your forehead.

Gene Fowler

To write a convincing paper, you must address many different questions,
ranging from the basics of who, what, when, where, why, and how, to whatever
additional questions and problems are raised during the dialogues that identify
and define your subject. How can you write a draft that covers all this?

We suggest in this chapter that you start by defining, organizing, and
planning the content; consider using techniques borrowed from successful
problem-solving strategies. Then learn the most effective ways of compiling the
information. After mastering basic word-processing skills, search out relevant
efficiency-enhancing features. Becoming adept at them will save much time in
the long run. Deal promptly with matters of authorship, both to minimize the
potential for misunderstandings and to guide collaboration and any division of
responsibility. Ease the writing task by paying attention to standard format
conventions. And finally, consider proven techniques to keep your writing
momentum going. Soon, your hardest work will be finished. You'll have
successfully completed a very effective first draft!

ORGANIZE AND PLAN THE CONTENT

All of us, when confronted by a writing deadline, face the temptation to skip the
organizational phases of writing. This is akin to leaving on a trip to unknown
parts without a road map! Professional writers are quick to point out that
organizing one's thoughts at the outset will save time in the long run, and will
result in a more effective document.

Whenever the subject of organization comes up, people picture an outline –
the most widely used technique for placing ideas in linear sequence for a written
document. However, organization has both a thinking and a writing stage, and
50% of any writing effort is taken by the thinking stage. At the thinking stage,
outlining is actually less effective than any of a number of other, lesser-known
activities, including brainstorming and clustering. You may wish to try out the
procedures mentioned below, and see which best contributes to the unity of
your document and eases the writing task.

If you find one or more of these techniques to be helpful, you will probably discover yourself using it freely and often. Some journalists use clustering to take notes during interviews, for example, developing a concept map as the responder talks. Technical writers report that these methods help minimize the edit–rewrite–edit–rewrite syndrome common in many commercial and academic situations. After capturing key points onto a concept map, issue tree, or cluster diagram, these writers translate the points into an organized list rather than a complete sentence draft. Only after approval of this version by supervisors do they go on to produce a full-sentence version.

To compile possibilities, consider brainstorming (random topic lists)

When you truly have no idea where to begin, try brainstorming. Brainstorming is a problem-solving technique in which one person or a group suggests as many ideas as possible about a given problem or situation, concentrating on quantity rather than quality; the result is a random topic list comprised of brief notes compiled quickly without much concern for order (Fig. 3.1).

Ideas on a brainstorming list often overlap. Some are general and some are specific. Some may be earthshaking, others silly. This is not only acceptable, but necessary and desirable. Avoid making judgments during this stage. This powerful idea-generating technique works best when the brain functions in an unrestricted manner.

After an exhaustive set of ideas has been listed on paper, evaluation and organization can begin. Use arrows or numbers to suggest an appropriate arrangement, such as chronological order or order of importance (see Table 3.1 on page 57). Consider the points in light of the potential audience, desired outcome, and publication constraints. Now the list can be rearranged, edited, and structured into a functional outline, if desired or required.

Things to mention about laryngeal neoplasia:

It's pretty rare.

It causes breathing troubles.

I'm glad I don't have it.

Radiographs usually show soft tissue masses.

Surgery is usually used to correct it.

It can be malignant or benign.

Surgical techniques should be described.

My patient recovered from it.

About 10 cases have been described from companion animals.

Fig. 3.1. A list compiled by brainstorming includes a variety of ideas.

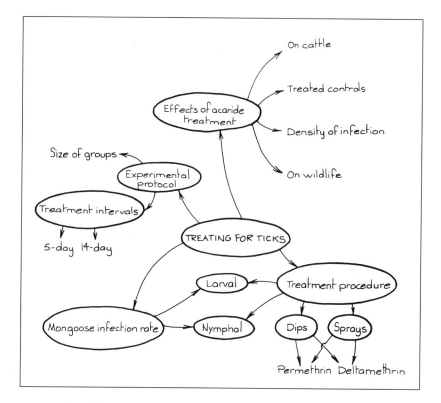

Fig. 3.2. The clustering process results in a type of concept map.

To suggest organization, try clustering (concept maps)

When you know what ideas you want to include, but are unsure about how to put them together, consider the technique called clustering. Midway in complexity between topic lists and outlining, this approach has been developed and refined more-or-less independently by various information-management experts in fields such as computer software development and data processing. As a result, the approach has many names and variations, but all involve a process – generally called clustering, brain writing, or branching – that results in weblike charts called concept maps, pattern notes, idea wheels, or bubble charts. For the visually oriented person, these charts can be an extremely effective way to organize information.

To begin clustering (Fig. 3.2), write the paper's main subject in the center of the page and circle it like the hub of a wheel. Think of major ways in which you could subdivide this subject, and write these ideas on the page at intervals around the circled main hub. Circle each of these second-level hubs (or bubbles, if you prefer that terminology), and draw lines or arrows connecting them to the central subject. Think about each of the second-level subjects. Near each one, add any details, examples, or further divisions. Circle these too, and draw lines connecting them to their respective subjects. Continue this process until you run out of ideas. When you see repetition, simply rearrange the pattern of spokes. If the pattern reaches the edge of the page, turn the spoke into another wheel hub, and start the process over to subdivide your ideas further.

After all of your ideas are clustered on the page, you may wish to go back and add numbers and letters to show the logical order. The numbered arrangement of these linked clusters can be used as a guide in organizing your writing and your final document.

To assess balance, develop an issue tree

An issue tree (Fig. 3.3) appears similar to an outline, and it looks more like the roots of a tree than its branches. These quibbles aside, an issue tree (Flower, 2000) can help check the balance of your treatment of a subject. More flexible than a formal outline, an issue tree is easy to rework during the organizing process and for a visually oriented person, it can seem less intimidating.

To develop an issue tree, write the main point at the top of a page. List

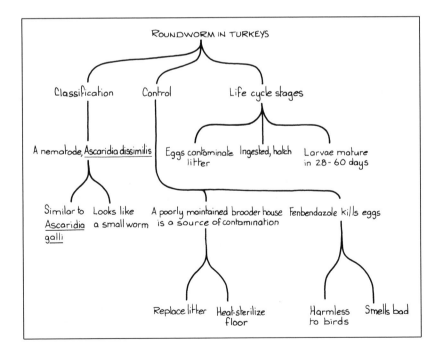

Fig. 3.3. An issue tree is a flexible tool for assessing balance in the treatment of a subject.

Table 3.1. *Common patterns for organizing material*

Pattern	Basis
Chronological	The sequence in which something happened
Geographical or spatial	The physical arrangement of entities
Functional	How parts work
Importance	Usually with elements in order of decreasing importance
Possible solutions	From least to most likely or best, or building to a climax
Specificity	General to particular, or particular to general
Complexity	Usually from simple to complex
Pro and con	Presenting both sides of an issue or decision
Causality	Cause and effect

subpoints under this main point. They may be phrased in any way that is comfortable, from single words to sentences or fragments. Then list subpoints below these, in decreasing order of importance. Connect all of these various levels with branching lines in a cascading manner.

As you explore topics, you may find that one branch begins to grow and spread across the page, almost excluding the others. Perhaps this material is an unnecessary digression. If so, this can be corrected at this early stage, before you have invested hours in drafting a narrative. Alternatively, the other branches may need more detail. Ask yourself questions about the subject of each branch: How do I know this? Why is it important? Does it contribute to the whole picture? What evidence do I have for this? Be as complete as you can.

To develop the paper's framework, consider an outline

Outlining is a time-honored technique, but it is important to remember that outlines serve two distinct purposes – to help organize one's thoughts, and to help organize one's written words. Some writers who find them useful for one of these purposes may find them less helpful for the other. Thus, the first decision should be whether to draw up an outline at all. You know your own personality best. If you decide to use an outline, the next decision is what kind.

Outlines come in many types, from sketchy affairs that are little more than lists to full-blown formal documents. Some extremely methodical writers first construct a topic outline to specify the order of the paper's sections, then develop a sentence outline to specify the order of the paragraphs within each section. Then and only then do they sit down to actually write. This is the time-honored formal outline system. Many of us subverted this process even back in English composition class, and wrote our required outlines only after the paper was finished. We either didn't know or didn't care that when we treated the outline as an afterthought, we negated most of its potential usefulness as an organizational tool. However, we did intuitively recognize that a working outline differs from a final writing outline, and only a masquerade could make them appear the same.

To discard the entire outlining process is to throw the baby out with the bath water, however. You may wish to consider developing an informal working outline, for your eyes only. In the early 1970s, a survey of members of the Society for Technical Communication found that 90% of those who responded used such a topic outline of words, phrases, and sentences. Only 5% used either a formal sentence outline or no outline at all. Likewise, some organizations require formal topical outlines for their publications.

Like the text of effective papers, strong formal outlines are filled with detail and established on a consistent pattern (Table 3.1). An outline structure can be developed that parallels the headings in the document, or vice versa.

Outlining is a fairly mechanical process, and most common word-processing programs have this capability. With automatic outlining, it will be dynamically updated each time the document is restructured. When the typescript is finished, this outline can be used to generate a table of contents and/or index, if needed. (Without an outline, headings still can be marked in the document so that a word-processing program can compile of table of contents from them. This is more tedious than the outline-based method, but it still is faster and more consistent than compiling such a table by hand.)

A typical topic outline consists of short phrases linked in a way that shows the sequential order and relative importance of ideas. The alphanumeric system (Fig. 3.4) alternates numbers and letters, and usually also uses degree of indention to indicate descending levels of headings.

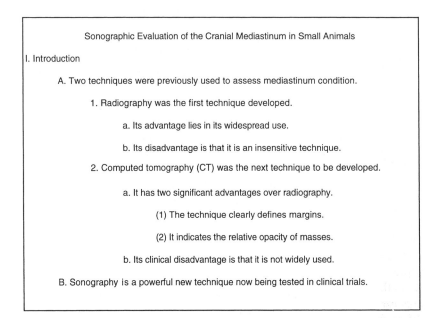

Fig. 3.4. An alphanumeric system is evident in this excerpt from a detailed, sentence-based outline.

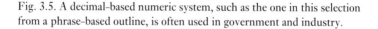

Pathogenicity of Two Field Strains of Infectious Bursal Disease Virus (IBDV)

1. (or 1.0). Description of IBDV

    1.1. Causative agent of Gumboro disease of young chickens

        1.11. Produces severe changes in Bursa of Fabricius

        1.12. Results in immunosuppression

    1.2. Classification

        1.21. Member of Birnavirus group

        1.22. Nonenveloped icosahedral virus

        1.23. Two serotypes (I and II)

2. (or 2.0). Timeliness of IBDV research

    3.1. IBD emergence as a major poultry disease problem

    3.2. Increase in subclinical IBD cases

    3.3. Many broiler farms losing money to this disease

Fig. 3.5. A decimal-based numeric system, such as the one in this selection from a phrase-based outline, is often used in government and industry.

Another type of outline is based on a numeric or decimal system (Fig. 3.5). Entries may be indented sequentially or all placed flush left. Decimal outlines are widely used in government and military publications. However, they can appear pretentious, and alphanumeric outlines are generally easier for readers to grasp.

Standard grammar books usually present specifically prescribed heading styles and rules of indentation. If your outline must pass outside review and critique, careful attention to such outlining conventions will help you gain approval. With either alphanumeric or numeric outlines, strive for consistency and balance. Use either complete sentences or just phrases or words, but never mix them. Each level also should always have two or more parts. If only one element appears, incorporate its information into the heading immediately above it.

DEAL WITH MATTERS OF AUTHORSHIP

Increasingly, scientific research involves collaboration, often across several disciplines. All contributors should receive credit for their particular contributions to the research, usually by being included as a coauthor. Joint authorship can be either a blessing or a curse, however, depending upon when and how it is approached.

Exercise 3–1. Organizing ideas

Reorganize the following outline of ideas, using a concept map or an issue tree. Compare your format with the examples given in Figs. 3.2 and 3.3.

ABUNDANCE OF SAND FLIES

A. Determining population dynamics
    1. Aspirating flies from resting sites
        a. 6 ft high tree holes (most were here)
        b. Ground level
    2. Light traps at different levels

B. Determining offspring age
    1. Laboratory studies
        a. Maximum age, 5 weeks
        b. 50% mortality by 2 weeks
    2. Field studies
        a. Most were 2–3 weeks old
        b. Youngest found, 1 week old

Discuss authorship before starting the first draft

Reach an explicit consensus on authorship as soon as you possibly can. Except possibly for the issue of plagiarism, nothing in the world of scientific publication is more likely to breed ill-will and wreck friendships than a disagreement over authorship.

Decisions on authorship should be guided by a simple ethical principle – any author listed on the paper's title page should take public responsibility for its content. No one should be an author unless they can take the responsibility for defending the paper's intellectual content. No one is likely to be able to take such responsibility unless they have taken part in the research *and* in writing the paper or revising it for accuracy of content.

Some individuals should *not* be included as coauthors – but often are. Participation solely in data collection or solely in the writing of the grant which funded the research does not necessarily justify authorship. Nor does general supervision of the laboratory group qualify one for authorship unless the supervisor contributed to the conception and design of the research or to the analysis and interpretation of the results. (Don't lose your job over this issue, however!)

Check the *Instructions to Authors*. Some *ITAs* require an explicit statement, signed by all the coauthors, to the effect that each author has contributed significantly to the paper, understands it, and endorses it. Further discussion of authorship can be found in the "Uniform Requirements for Manuscripts Submitted to Biomedical Journals" (Appendix 2).

Agree on the order of authors' names

Why does it matter in what order names appear on the title page of a typescript or published paper? One reason is that the order implies the authors' relative contributions. The first name to appear is generally assumed to be the individual who played the largest part in the study. This person is called the senior author. In some laboratories, the head of the laboratory, department, or research team is automatically included on any paper coming from the laboratory, often as senior author but sometimes as the second or even last-listed author.

Visibility is a second reason. If several people have worked together on a project, and you are not one of the first three authors named, be prepared for your name to be invisible in other authors' articles. In reference lists (and sometimes in text as well), journals typically print all the names up to some arbitrary number (three or six are common choices). Beyond this number, they usually include only the first one or three names, and use *et al.* for the rest.

When many people all have contributed more or less equally to the research, alphabetical or reverse alphabetical name order is sometimes used. Alternatively, if more than one paper logically comes from a cooperative project, authors sometimes rotate as first author on successive publications.

Many research reports result from the efforts of large cooperative teams. (Perhaps a record for the greatest number of coauthors on a single publication is the 488 individuals from 39 institutions for an article in *Physical Particle Physics*!) Although authors generally would like to see their individual names appear, when this many people are involved, editors may like to see authorship credited by group titles. Rather than listing the names of individuals, none of whom can really take responsibility for the whole, the group could coin a designation, such as "The National Cooperative Atherosclerosis Study." A footnote would list group members, and each could legitimately list the paper on their personal résumés.

Let authorship guide collaboration, and vice versa

An early decision about authorship allows the work of writing to be divided accordingly. When several people are collaborating on a typescript, one's first temptation may be to simply assign a section to each, then compile the sections. This poses potential problems – including illogical strategy, weak transitions, and inconsistencies in language, to name a few of the more common.

An alternative method of dividing responsibility that often works better is to designate the best writer in the group as coordinator. Assign this person the responsibility for the outline, introduction, summary, and conclusions. Divide responsibility for the other sections among the remaining authors. Set clear deadlines for each step of the writing. Communicate often and clearly, using email for speed and efficiency if possible.

When the rough drafts are collected, give the coordinator the license to change any section in order to make it flow smoothly into the whole. Then give all contributors the opportunity to comment on a revised draft. Before submitting the final version to a journal, be sure to have all coauthors read and approve it.

UNDERSTAND MATTERS OF COPYRIGHT

Copyright is the right of exclusive ownership by an author of the benefits resulting from the creation of his or her work. It covers the matter and form of a literary or artistic work, i.e., how it is expressed. It does not cover the ideas or data themselves, but just the way in which they have been presented.

Copyright gives authors (or others to whom they transfer copyright ownership) control over how the work is reproduced and disseminated. Once copyrighted, a work cannot be indiscriminately reproduced unless the copyright owner gives permission, usually in exchange for royalties or other compensation.

The issue of copyright affects both your use of others' work and your own published writing. Publications that explain the copyright law in detail are available from the Copyright Office, Library of Congress, Washington, DC 20559.

Determine whether published material is copyrighted

A work first published after March 1, 1989, receives copyright protection whether or not it bears a notice of copyright. However almost all published materials generally contain such a notice, usually on the back of the title page. In fact, this is often called the "copyright page." If a book was published after January 1, 1978, the term of the copyright is for the author's life plus 50 years. If it was published before 1978, the first copyright term covers 28 years, but it is renewable for an additional 47 years.

All publications created by U.S. government agencies are in the public domain. That is, they are not copyrighted, and may be used freely.

Understand "fair use"

Copyright law provides a "fair use" provision that allows others such as teachers, librarians, and reviewers to reproduce a limited portion of copyrighted materials for educational and certain other purposes without compensation to the copyright owners. The law refers to such purposes as "criticism, comment, news reporting, teaching (including multiple copies for classroom use), scholarship or research." The fair use provision does not allow you to copy complete articles and republish them without permission, even if it is not done for profit.

A small amount of material from a copyrighted source may be used in your written work without permission or payment as long as the use satisfies the fair use criteria and is not harmful to the rights of the copyright owner. However, you always should give credit to the source from which the material was taken.

With the advent of the Internet, many copyrighted works formerly available solely in print are now distributed around the world in cyberspace. Copyright law applies to cyberspace works just as it does to their print counterparts. Even if the fair use provision applies to your intended use of such materials, their source must be documented. If you plan to reproduce or further distribute copyrighted works available on the Internet beyond the fair use provision, you must first obtain permission from the copyright holder.

Understand how copyright affects your own publication

When you write a scientific research paper, you own the copyright for the length of your life plus 50 years, unless it was done for an employer or commissioned as work for hire. If you have coauthors, each of you is a co-owner of the copyright, with equal rights.

When you publish this paper in a journal, copyright is generally transferred to the publisher, who will handle such paperwork as filing the copyright application and responding to future requests to use the material. Before the Copyright Act of 1976, this transfer usually happened somewhat automatically. Now, it must be specifically written out, so most publishers ask authors to sign a copyright transfer form.

If work to which you hold copyright is to be published in electronic format, be sure to fully investigate your rights under current copyright law. Publishers and authors are banding together to identify and manage this new and rapidly changing area, through such systems as Publisher Item Identifier (PII). This tagging system for both print and electronic formats is used by the American Chemical Society and the American Mathematical Society, among others (Day, 1998). The copyright owner of a published work can generate its PII tag.

If for some reason you are interested in securing copyright on a book or manuscript yourself, information can be obtained from the Register of Copyright, Copyright Office, Library of Congress, Washington, DC 20559.

FOLLOW STANDARD STRUCTURE

By this point in life, you've undoubtedly seen enough scientific documents to recognize that almost all of them follow a quite similar pattern. Each main section is structured to address certain questions, and together they shape a critical argument. This is the accepted format for publication in a scientific journal, and should not be changed without an extremely good reason.

Happily, this fairly rigid structure usually makes scientific writing easier, not more difficult. The next few pages offer a brief overview of what will be required. When you plunge in and begin to write, refer back here as necessary for inspiration and to stay on track.

Introduction – What is the problem and why should anyone care?

Why was this work done? Deal with the question briefly, interestingly, and as simply as possible. A well-written Introduction should persuade colleagues and even non-specialists to begin reading the paper's text once their attention has been attracted by the title, abstract, tables, and figures.

A three-part Introduction works well. First state the general field of interest. Concisely present what is already known about the subject of your investigation, referencing the most important publications. Don't try to mention everything, unless you are writing a review article or a thesis. One to three paragraphs should be enough for most journal articles.

Next, present others' findings that will be challenged or expanded. Explain how you are hoping to extend or modify what is already known or believed. Provide support for your argument.

Finally, specify the question which the paper addresses, and how it does so. This sentence is often phrased in hypothesis form. Indicate your experimental approach. Point out what is new and important about your work. When appropriate, briefly summarize the answer(s) you found.

Materials and Methods – How was the evidence obtained?

This section may have any of several names – Materials and/or Methods, Experimental Design, Protocol, and Procedure are some of the common ones. Sometimes it is divided into separately titled subsections, as well.

Begin with necessary supplies, including both animate materials such as experimental animals and inanimate ones such as chemicals. Explicitly note that use of animals and human subjects conformed to the legal requirements for the country in which the research was conducted. Next, specify what was done, and for what purpose. Chronological order is a common way to proceed through this segment. Alternatively, parallel the sequence in which you present results. A flow chart may be useful for readers. Conclude with a discussion of any statistical procedures employed (but not the tests' outcomes, which belong in Results).

The key to a successful Methods section is to include the right amount of detail – too much, and it begins to sound like a laboratory manual; too little, and no one can repeat what was done. As an additional guide, frequently refer to examples published in the chosen journal. For publication of a new discovery to be "valid" (see pages 5–6) or scientifically accepted, it must appear in a form so that a reader could repeat the experiment. However, this really means not just any reader, but a trained investigator with considerable experience. Once again, it is important to know one's audience.

Increasingly, federally funded research in the United States is requiring studies to be conducted in accordance with Good Laboratory Practice (GLP) guidelines (Benson and Boege, 1999). The guidelines require preparation of standard operating procedures for all aspects of a project. Referring back to these procedures can be very helpful when preparing Materials and Methods and when documenting the data which were collected. Even when GLP guidelines are not required for a project, using this research approach facilitates the writing task.

Don't use the Methods to reinvent the wheel. If you have followed a widely known method, simply name the principles on which it is based and cite the original publication or recent textbooks or handbooks that give full details. If you made changes to a published procedure, describe only the changes and reference the rest. Only if you have employed an entirely new process or technique must you describe it in full. In this last instance, you may wish to test the adequacy of your description by asking a colleague to do an experiment using the technique as your typescript describes it (Booth, 1993).

Results – What was found or seen?

This section should be relatively easy. Decide on a logical order for presentation (see Table 3.1 on page 57). One style is to present the most important results first. Another is to go from simple results to complex ones. Still another way is to present data in a chronological order that parallels the way the methods were applied during the study.

Present the results that have a bearing on the question you are examining, but do not interpret them here; defer that task to the Discussion section. Exclude irrelevant findings, but never omit valid results that appear to contradict your hypothesis. Suppressing such data is unethical, but when presenting them you may explain why you feel they are anomalous.

Tables and figures are usually an integral part of this section. Don't use the text to parrot the information they contain. Readers can see the data for themselves. Instead, point out salient features and relationships between the various results.

Discussion and Conclusion – What do these findings mean?

These sections, often combined with each other and sometimes with the Results as well, are the place to answer the specific question or questions stated in the Introduction. Their organization may parallel that used in earlier sections of the paper. Often, the most salient findings are presented first.

This is the place to interpret your results against a background of existing knowledge. Explain what is new in your work, and why it matters. Discuss both the limitations and the implications of your results, and relate observations to other relevant studies. State new hypotheses when warranted, clearly labeled as such. Include recommendations, when appropriate.

When writing this section, watch for symptoms of megalomania. Avoid exaggerated or extravagant claims for your work, and carefully distinguish between facts and speculation. Be wary about extrapolating your results to other species or conditions. When discussing other results and hypotheses that are relevant to yours, be tactful about apparent disagreements. Particularly, rein in the natural human tendency to want to point out the shortcomings of another investigator's report. Indicate what the next steps might be to resolve any apparent conflicts. Frankly admit anomalies. Discuss any possible errors or limitations in your methods and assumptions. And finally, don't stack in so many alternative hypotheses to explain the results that readers become buried in the pile.

The title – What is the paper about?

From the moment when the first words are written, every document needs a rough working title for identification purposes. One of us keeps a running list of possible titles throughout the development of a typescript, tucked away in the "reservoir" notebook (see pages 3–4).

However, working titles are rarely suitable for the final paper. After drafting the main sections of the paper, it is time to refine the title. Is it interesting, concise, and informative? Is it accurate enough for use in indexing systems and bibliographic databases? Remember, many readers will judge your paper's relevance to their own interests on the basis of the title alone.

Most journals prefer short titles, typically not over 100 characters, including the spaces between the words. This generally works out to only 10–12 words. Check the target journal at the outset; some limit titles even more drastically. Keep the title length down by cutting out trivial phrases (such as "Notes on" or "A study of"), but do not use uncommon abbreviations or stack nouns and adjectives together without the prepositions that clarify their meaning.

> *Poor:* A Study of Chipmunk Muscle Tissue Ion Channel Amino Acid Activation Parameters
>
> *Better:* Amino Acid Activation of Ion Channels in Chipmunk Muscle Tissue

A poor title may not scuttle a paper's chances of publication, but it certainly can start one off on the wrong foot with editors. Examine past issues of the journal for insights. In general, editors frown upon misleading or fanciful titles. Many ban titles that make claims about the findings in the paper (but a few encourage them by example). Some also object to two-part titles, with a main title and a subtitle. Titles that end with a question mark are seldom acceptable.

> *Risky choices:* Pollen Between a Rock and a Hard Place: German and Austrian Saxifrages
>
> Does *Saxifraga* Pollen in Germany Resemble That in Austria?
>
> German Saxifrage Pollens are Superior to Those in Austria
>
> *Safer choice:* Pollen Morphology of German and Austrian *Saxifraga* Species

You may be writing a series of papers on a subject, but title each one separately. Numbered series with the same title and differing subtitles are nothing but a headache to everyone, especially if they have slightly different sets of coauthors. Journals are unhappy with the implication that acceptance of one paper obligates them to publish successive ones. Readers, librarians, and cataloguers have to deal with unnecessary confusion, especially if part 4 is published before part 2, or part 3 is rejected entirely. If you feel it is vital that everyone knows the papers are a series, link them by mentioning the others in a footnote on the title page or by citing them in the Introduction. (Remember that if the typescript on hand is interdependent with another paper that is either unsubmitted or unpublished, include copies of that other paper for reviewers when you send the typescript to an editor.)

References – Who did what?

There are literally hundreds of variations of literature reference schemes, and some excellent computerized bibliographic programs are available to help you consistently apply proper formatting to your final draft. For now, the most important task is to keep text material properly linked to its attribution. Regardless of the journal's reference style, consider using the name–and–year system (also called the Harvard system) rather than consecutive numbers for references in the first draft. It is easier to compile a final reference list from names than from numbers, and minimizes the chances that reference citations will become scrambled during reorganizations of the text.

Note that some journals limit the number of references you can cite; check the *Instructions to Authors*. One common restriction is 40 references for full articles and 10 for brief communications, but some journals specify even fewer.

Abstracts and Summaries are different entities

Athough some journals use the term "summary" to describe abstracts of their articles, a summary is not the same as an abstract. An abstract is an abbreviated version of the paper, written for people who may never read the complete version. A summary restates the main findings and conclusions of a paper, and is written for people who have already read the paper. Include a summary only if the journal requires it.

Abstracts come in several varieties, and examples in the journal will demonstrate what is required. By definition, an abstract strives to provide an abbreviated but accurate representation of the contents of a document, without added interpretation or criticism and without distinction as to who wrote it.

Informative abstracts include some data, and are commonly used with documents that describe original research. They address the same questions as the body of the paper, but briefly and without supporting tables or figures. Indicative abstracts are descriptive, containing general statements about the subjects covered. They are often used for review articles or books. Both informative and indicative abstracts are typically limited to between 100 and 250 words, and different points are emphasized in proportion to the emphasis they receive in the text itself. They are generally written as a single paragraph.

Structured abstracts are often longer, sometimes allowing as many as 400 words. These abstracts group series of points below headings such as Objective,

Design, Setting, Patients, Treatment, Results, Conclusions, and Clinical Relevance. Experts disagree whether structured abstracts are on the way to disappearance or are evolving into a new kind of publication, with the main text available only in electronic form.

Staying within an abstract's word count specifications is a challenge for almost every writer. The title and abstract are always read together, so there is no reason to waste words by repeating or paraphrasing the title in the abstract. Be as brief and specific as possible, but write complete sentences that logically follow one another. Use the third person, active verbs, and the past tense unless it becomes unacceptably awkward to do so.

Regardless of its form, an abstract must be written so it can stand on its own merits without the text (which many readers will never see). For this reason, one should generally avoid citing others' work in an abstract; if a citation is essential, however, include a short form of the bibliographic details in the abstract itself. Likewise, it is best to avoid unfamiliar terms, acronyms, abbreviations, or symbols; if they must be used, define them at first mention in the abstract, then again at first mention in the text. And finally, never introduce information in the abstract that is not covered in the paper.

Attend to the title page, keywords, acknowledgments, and the rest

To complete the first draft, review the *Instructions to Authors* for the intended journal for any other sections that may be required. These commonly include a title page with a suggested running head, keywords, and acknowledgments.

The title page really doesn't need to be compiled until the final draft is assembled. However, for a psychological sense of completeness, writers often like to put one on the first draft. Furthermore, drafting this page now allows coauthors to check such fundamentals as the spelling of their names and the accuracy of their institutional affiliations. Most journals specify what other information should appear on this page. Commonly it includes authors' degrees, job titles, and the name and addresses (postal and electronic) of the author to whom correspondence, proofs, and requests for reprints should be sent. Keywords and funding sources also may appear here.

Keywords or key phrases are intended as indexing and cataloguing entries. They commonly appear either before or after the abstract. In some journals, keywords are displayed with the titles in the table of contents. The number of keywords that can be included is usually specified; three to ten are common limits, but check the *Instructions to Authors*.

If guidance from the journal is lacking, it is generally prudent to choose keywords and terms from the Medical Subject Headings used in *Index Medicus*, or from lists such as those published in *Biological Abstracts* and *Chemical Abstracts*. Choose the most important and most specific terms you can find in your document, including more general terms only if your work has interdisciplinary significance. Unless the target journal specifies otherwise, words that appear in the title do not need to be included among the keywords.

Acknowledgments should be brief and straightforward. (Note that some journals spell the title of this section with two *e*s, others with three.) Include any substantial help received from organizations or individuals, whether they provided grants, materials, technical assistance, or advice. (Some journals specify that funding bodies be named on the title page instead.) Thank those who went out of their way to help, but not people who did not contribute directly to the reported work or those who did no more than their routine laboratory or office work. Some *Instructions to Authors* explicitly state, "do not acknowledge editorial or secretarial help." Others require signed permissions from everyone who is acknowledged.

Exercise 3–2. Title choices

How could the following manuscript titles be improved? Explain the reasons for your choices.

1. Plantar's Wart Removal: Report of a Case of Recurrence of Verruca after Curative Excision

2. Characteristics of Columbine Flowers are Correlated with Their Pollinators

3. Panda Mating Fails: Veterinarian Takes Over

4. Gleanings On The Bionomics And Behavior Of The East Asiatic Nonsocial Wasps. III. The Subfamily Crabroninae With A Key To The Species Of The Tribe Crabronini Occurring In Formosa And The Ryukyus, Contributions To The Knowledge Of The Behavior Of Crabronine Fauna, And Changes In The Taxonomic Position Of Three Species Of Crabronini Occurring In Japan

5. Report of New Health Data Results from the 1999 National ASAP-FYI-ERGO Health Study: Lung Cancer in Women Mushrooms

---

APPROACH WRITING IN A WAY THAT BUILDS
MOMENTUM – AND KEEPS IT

> There ain't no rules around here! We're trying to accomplish something!
> *Thomas Edison*

Ready to begin "really" writing? It's time to work with – not against – your natural habits, for you'll find that the key to success is building up a head of steam with a steady sense of progress that propels you on toward completion.

Start in the place that makes sense for you

When it comes to writing style, are you basically a rabbit or a turtle? As Michael Alley (1987) explains:

Rabbits hate first drafts. They hate juggling audience and research with all the elements of style. In a first draft, they sprint; they write down everything and anything. They use pens – no time for erasing – and their pens never leave the paper. Rabbits strap themselves to the chair and will not get up for anything. Rabbits finish drafts quickly, but their early drafts are horrendous, many times not much better than their outlines. Nonetheless, they've got something. They've got their ideas on paper, and they're in a position to revise.   Alley (1987), p. 195

Turtles are quite the opposite. They patiently accept the job before them, and work through it methodically:

A turtle tries not to write down a sentence unless it's perfect. In the first sitting, a turtle begins with one sentence and slowly builds on that sentence with another, then another. In the second sitting, a turtle . . . revises everything from the first sitting before adding on. It usually takes a turtle several sittings to finish a first draft, but the first draft is strong . . . the beginning and middle are usually very tight because they've been reworked so many times. Revision usually entails smoothing the ending as well as checking the overall structure.
                                                Alley (1987), pp. 195–196

Few writers are strictly one or the other, of course, but you'll be most efficient if you determine which approach best fits your general style and personality. If you have turtle tendencies, ease into the first draft by starting with the section you feel is the most straightforward. (For many people, it is Materials and Methods.) If you are a rabbit type, begin with the Introduction and just plow right on, quickly getting as much information written as possible.

Set a realistic goal for each sitting. Don't stop until you've reached it, even if you become pressed for time and must "cheat" by finishing the section in outline form. Reaching a goal is almost guaranteed to give you a feeling of accomplishment that will help keep your momentum going. But don't stop here. Before you finish, write a few sentences of the next section. Psychologically, this makes it easier to start writing next time. Some writers claim it even helps to stop in mid-sentence or mid-thought!

Minimize distractions any way you can

While you are writing, it is worth making the effort to remove or escape from as many distractions as possible. Because each sentence in a scientific paper depends so much upon those around it, losing momentum usually leads to losing one's train of thought. Try to find a time and place when you can be relatively undisturbed.

Inevitably, from time to time your thoughts will tend to fly off in surprising directions while you are immersed in your work. Don't try to remember one set of ideas while working on another. They will either sidetrack you, or flutter off and never be recaptured. Keep a note pad near your work. Pen unrelated ideas onto a list when they occur, and deal with them later.

Watch what you eat. This tip may seem frivolous to those who have never been involved in a really lengthy writing project. However, as Alley (1987) points out, writing makes people restless, which often makes them hungry. The wrong choice of snacks can derail your writing momentum. If you must eat, choose foods that require only one hand, don't stain papers, and don't make you thirsty or (worse yet) sleepy.

Keep the text simple, but somewhat organized

Write as simply as possible. Remember those readers who will not be specialists in your area of research, and may not be reading in their native language. Imagine that you are describing your work to an interested friend in another scientific discipline. At this stage, don't worry too much about details of style or grammar, however. These things can be fixed at the revision stage.

Readers need a story line – a beginning, a middle, and an end, with clear links between each step. Insert headings to guide the way, especially if the paper is long. Follow your outline or other organizational aid, but treat it as a life jacket, not a straitjacket. As you write, new insights may come to mind and some previously identified topics may become irrelevant.

When really pressed for time, spend more time on the first draft, not less

A caveat is in order here. When you are in a hurry, be conservative. Take the extra time to develop a first-draft structure your coauthors or other readers can easily follow. Work steadily and quickly, and get the whole thing on paper in as rational an arrangement as you can. There may be no time to cut, paste, and rearrange. There may not even be time to polish. It's admittedly a horrible thought, but it would be even more horrible to have the paper in bits and pieces when the clock strikes!

Write around missing information

A common cause of lost momentum is the missing word. It's on the tip of your tongue, but after 5 minutes spent looking in the dictionary you still can't find it, and you've ground to a halt as a result. Write the name of your favorite sports team, your significant other, or simply "???" in its place, and keep on going. Your subconscious will bring it to the surface later. When that happens, don't forget to use the "search and replace" command in your word-processing program to find your space-holder and insert the word where it belongs.

If you can't find the sentence to express an idea, you may not have fully formed the idea yet. Again, leave a space-holder, and keep on writing. Think about it later, perhaps when you are exerting yourself physically; many writers and researchers feel that exercise sharpens their processing of ideas.

Recognize the signs of bogging down

At some point in the writing process, you may feel overwhelmed. It can be an intense emotion, but be reassured that most writers experience these feelings as a very natural reaction to the magnitude of their task. Words rarely flow effortlessly all the time for anyone. Professional writers struggle, just like you do. Everyone also experiences times when their writing efficiency seems to decline or die.

Instead of quitting altogether when such feelings strike, switch to writing a different section. Alternatively, begin to write (or talk) about precisely why you are bogged down – surprisingly, this exercise often will free you. If you stop when you are stalled, it can become an excuse to avoid starting up again.

Deal constructively with writer's block

It's a writer's worst fear. The deadline is fast approaching. You sit down to write and absolutely nothing useful happens . . . You chew your pencil or tap a rhythm on the computer console, stare out the window, get up for a drink of water, decide to run an errand or shop for groceries . . . . The inspiration to write has vanished. You have writer's block. Or do you?

Those who write about writing debate whether writer's block is a real phenomenon or just a bit of folklore used to explain garden-variety distraction and provide an excuse to stop working. Whatever may ultimately be decided, a great number of solutions fortunately have been suggested. Many of them sound like the ideas we've already mentioned. Here are a few other imaginative suggestions:

> Alley (1987) believes that writer's block can arise because many of us are inhibited by hidden voices, such as criticism from our eighth grade English teacher or our department manager. He suggests drowning them out with classical or jazz music.
>
> Even when you can't get a word down on paper, Shortland and Gregory (1991) point out that you might find that you could easily talk to friends about your topic. Write down what you would say, much in the manner of a rambling letter to a close friend. (Or, as a colleague suggests, record your conversation, and listen to it for ideas.) It will become easier to keep going once you have words on paper instead of still in your mind, and you may even make your story more understandable to your audience than it would other-wise be.
>
> For particularly severe cases, Mack and Skjei (1979) recommend a technique called "kitchen-sinking it," in which one repeatedly sits down and writes nonstop for a fixed but short time (such as 15 minutes) about any aspect of the paper's topic. One ends up with "everything but the kitchen sink," but these bits can be revised and pieced together for a first draft. It may be crude but it is a

start, and this is often enough to get the writing process flowing once again. Reading over this mixture helps promote a focus on ideas.

In an interesting turnaround, Nelson (1993) suggests that rather than treating the symptoms, an author should view writer's block as an asset – the creative mind's healthy response to an inner imbalance – and use it as a stepping stone to new levels of creativity and artistic growth. Presenting writer's block as a constellation of problems with different causes and treatments, Nelson offers ideas tailored to such situations as beginner's block, perfectionism, notes and plans that refuse to make a book, and obsessive rewriting.

Perhaps the most important defense against writer's block is simply to keep in mind that a first draft is a first draft. It will not go to the editor, the typescript consultants, the printer, your department head, or perhaps not even the coauthors. You are the only one who ever needs to see it. A first draft will have intellectual faults and flaws in prose. You will have many chances to correct these later. Instead of worrying about its imperfections, congratulate yourself. With the first draft in hand, you have successfully completed the hardest parts of scientific writing! Now, if at all possible, set it aside to "cool" a bit, and go work on something else.

4

Supporting the text with tables and figures

Art, like morality, consists of drawing the line somewhere.

G. K. Chesterton

Whether or not one is prepared to call them art, the visual aids that are included in most scientific papers can be vitally important in presenting the scientist's message. They summarize and emphasize key points and reduce narrative length. They simplify information, thus enhancing understanding. They improve the conciseness and clarity of the narrative. And finally, when carefully crafted, they add visual appeal to a manuscript.

Readers often look at tables and figures to see whether the rest of a paper is worth reading, and while they may not go on to read every sentence, they almost always look at every illustration. Each must contribute an essential part to the text, and each must be capable of standing on its own without reference to the text.

Because tables and figures both present data in condensed form and help clarify and support ideas, they function as a time-saving writing tool. In our experience, the earlier one starts preparing them, the better. Designing graphics early in the writing process can minimize the amount of writing, saving hours of drafting and editing time.

CHOOSE VISUAL AIDS WISELY AND USE THEM WELL

To an editor, every visual aid is an illustration, and every illustration that isn't a table is a figure. Tables are the most used (and many say, overused) form of illustration in scientific writing. Figures include a tremendous variety of other text accompaniments, including line graphs, histograms, maps, photographs, and drawings. Each type has its own strengths and weaknesses, but all deserve more attention from researchers and writers than they currently receive.

Is this illustration really necessary?

Any use of documentary illustrations should begin with this question. Too often, scientists thoughtlessly include excessive illustrations, merely because they have them. Often a line or two of text would give the same information far more economically. Do readers really need to see the trace made by a graphic recorder pen? Do they need to see a "typical" chicken afflicted with a well-known disease? Sometimes it seems as though visual aids have been included only to prove the research occurred. ("See, it really *did* happen like I said it did!")

Choose the illustration that best fits the purpose

Many illustrations transform numerical data into other shapes. Graphs and histograms are examples. Developing these visual aids takes more conscious effort than tables do, but they are often the most powerful way to express relationships. They can illuminate ideas and trends that would be all but invisible to readers if the same data were presented in conventional table form.

Other types of illustrations present primary evidence of the scientific observations. Instrument tracings, photographs, and micrographs document the material presented in the text. Sometimes they are literally "worth a thousand words" but in other cases they can be blatantly irrelevant to a paper's message.

Another category includes explanatory materials such as maps, charts, line drawings, and "gazintas" (see page 95). The less familiar with your work your potential audience is expected to be, the more strongly you should consider including illustrations of this type.

The brief checklist given in Table 4.1 can help you determine which types of illustration will be the most appropriate for a particular purpose. In this chapter, we'll examine effective ways to use these different types of illustrative materials. Helpful sources of additional information include Briscoe (1996), Brock (1990), and Council of Biology Editors (1988).

Suit the illustration to the audience

Deciding which illustration format would be most appropriate or most informative is not only a matter of its purpose. One's scientific discipline, the particular data set, and the intended journal and audience will also influence this decision.

For example, from time to time you may be called upon to make an oral presentation to colleagues, managers, or administrators, or a general audience outside your special area of expertise. Nearly every such presentation uses some type of visual aid, traditionally the most popular being the 35-mm slide, followed by overhead transparencies, flipcharts, films, videotapes, and even filmstrips and the old schoolroom standard, the chalkboard or markerboard. Increasingly, such presentations are being computerized, and several excellent supporting software programs now exist.

Communicating your work to others outside your area of expertise can be a challenge, but it is one we urge you to accept, for the rewards can be great. This is your opportunity to present your message to a broad and receptive audience. Do not bore or alienate them by reading your speech, report, or technical paper. Instead, talk to them. Tell them what is interesting and important about your subject. Stress the high points.

Table 4.1. *Choosing the most effective type of illustration for a given goal*

To accomplish this	Choose one of these
To present exact values, raw data, or data which do not fit into any simple pattern	Table, list
To summarize trends, show interactions between two or more variables, relate data to constants, or emphasize an overall pattern rather than specific measurements	Line graph
To dramatize differences or draw comparisons	Bar graph
To illustrate complex relationships, spatial configurations, pathways, processes, or interactions	Diagram
To show sequential processes	Flowchart
To classify information	Table, list, pictograph
To describe parts or electric circuits	Schematic
To describe a process, organization, or model	Pictograph, flowchart, block diagram
To compare or contrast	Pictograph, pie chart, bar graph
To describe a change of state	Line graph, bar graph
To describe proportions	Pie chart, bar graph
To describe relationships	Table, line graph, block diagram
To describe causation	Flowchart, pictograph
To describe an entire object	Schematic, drawing, photograph
To show the vertical or horizontal hierarchy within an object, idea, or organization	Flowchart, drawing tree, block diagram

Whether in print or oral presentation, a cordial and competent approach underscored with lighthearted visual aids goes a long way in warming a lay audience to your cause. Never talk down to an audience, but don't be afraid to use analogies and humor. And, always illustrate your dialogue with the most appropriate and effective illustrations you can design. Many things are communicated better in pictures than in words. For greatest effectiveness, use simple graphics, and make each illustrate a single point. Include a minimum of labels, and put them on the drawings rather than in a separate legend. Investigate any size restraints which may govern the illustration's final form.

Do not simply borrow material designed for journal publication. An illustration prepared for one medium seldom works effectively in another. An audience of kennel club members will not appreciate a table showing canine ocular fluid pressure values expressed to three decimal points that was quite appropriate for a specialized journal. A visually attractive graph presenting trends and relationships would be better received.

Information that will be presented on a display board, slide, or overhead transparency should be prepared with their purpose in mind. For a fast-paced talk at a research meeting, simple tables showing small amounts of numerical data would be desirable as visual aids, whereas numerically complex tables might be overwhelming. In a written document, however, the same information might be summarized in the text or included within larger, more complex tables to be examined by the reader in a more leisurely fashion.

Check journal requirements

Because illustrations cost more to reproduce than text, some publications strictly regulate their number, size, and type. Knowing this at the outset can save a lot of time; check *Instructions to Authors* and format in the journal itself. Reduce the odds of editorial requests for last-minute revision by not pushing the limits unnecessarily.

As a useful general rule, a scientific manuscript should include no more than one table or illustration per 1000 words of text. This can be easily determined with the word count feature of a word-processing program. As a rough estimate, the average page of text in a manuscript that is typed double spaced with one-inch margins has between 200 and 250 words. Therefore, the guideline might be stated as no more than one table or illustration per four pages of manuscript text.

Some journals accept only tables and line drawings (such as diagrams and graphs). Others also accept black-and-white photographs, which are then photographed again through a screen grid to produce dots that make up a printed image called a half-tone. Half-tones are usually of lesser quality than the originals because the printing process may transfer the image several times with some loss of clarity at each transfer.

Some scientific journals will not print color photographs. A few will accept them only if the author agrees to pay some or all of the reproduction cost, which is usually high. Black-and-white prints can be made from color photographs or transparencies, but their quality will suffer. Whenever possible, it is better to start with a black-and-white photograph in the first place. Digital camera images yield good color or black and white prints.

Make each illustration independent but integral

Paradoxically, good tables and figures should both stand alone and be an indispensable part of the text.

A reader should be able to understand each illustration without referring to the text. For this, the title must be adequate, the headings complete and explanatory, and the data arranged logically. The text, in turn, must refer specifically to each table and figure by number and clarify why the information is needed. The standard "Table 1 gives results" falls short in this regard, and simply wastes space. Use the text to summarize or explain, as in "Affected animals had significantly lower weights (Table 1)."

Consider the set of tables and other illustrations in a document as a sequence. Together, they should tell a story – the message of the paper. However, avoid saying "as shown in the table above/below" because the position and page number of a table is not determined until typesetting by the printer.

Label illustrations carefully and completely

This advice may seem premature, but because illustrations tend to be stored and processed separately from text, they can become separated from a manuscript during handling and are particularly vulnerable to loss, a costly situation in both time and dollars.

As soon as an illustration is prepared, place a label on the back side to identify it with your name, address, article or report title, and a unique identifying number. Because a few journals do not accept adhesive labels (especially for color photographs), check the *Instructions to Authors* and follow directions, if any, for labeling illustrative materials. To avoid the embarrassment of an incorrectly oriented figure, include the word *top*, accompanied by an arrow. Never write on the illustration itself; the writing can show through on the front.

Place figures in a separate oversized envelope, and label the envelope with your name and a short title for the paper. Keep any original artwork and at least one duplicate set of all illustrations.

USE TABLES TO PRESENT COMPLEX DATA OR PARALLEL DESCRIPTIONS

Everyone has seen scientific tables. They range from informal in-text presentations hardly more complicated than a word list to complex formal compilations spanning several pages. Tables are, in fact, the single most overused form of visual aid in scientific writing. Their use is so widespread in most scientific and technical fields that some beginning writers judge them to be an indispensable part of every scientific paper. Although most of us find tables to be the easiest graphic aid to compile, they are not necessarily appropriate for every paper.

In the process of conducting research we tend to rough out tables to consolidate data, or to summarize relevant information. The urge can be overwhelming to import these tables wholesale into the document. Resist this temptation. The fact that a table has been a useful organizational tool is not sufficient justification for its automatic inclusion in the text. Nor should numerical data be included solely because they were collected. Every study involves a certain amount of effort spent in gathering data that later turn out not to be needed. Careful planning can minimize this fact, but never eliminate it entirely. Have the courage to prune extraneous material.

At some point between the first draft and the final manuscript, make a concerted effort to decide which tables might be combined, which tables would be better replaced by other illustrative materials, and which tables should be discarded in favor of summarizing the data in the text.

Word tables and numerical tables have their place

All this having been said, we must stress that tables are sometimes the best illustrations for a scientific paper. Word tables present parallel descriptions concisely. In medical writing, tables that appear in case series analyses provide a good example of their appropriate use. In an oral presentation, a teaching article, or a review, small tables of text (which function like figures) also may be used to emphasize the main points or included as a handy reference like the example in Table 4.2.

Table 4.2. *A helpful word table: Cloned human gene products*

Protein	Used in treating
Insulin	Diabetes
Growth hormone	Pituitary dwarfism
Erythropoietin	Anemia
Factor VIII	Hemophilia
Interleukin-2	Cancer
Tissue plasminogen factor	Heart attack, stroke

Numerical tables provide a compact way of presenting complex information in a format that invites comparisons that would be lost or incomprehensible in narrative form. A useful rule of thumb (Bjelland, 1990) is to use a table when putting data in the text would take at least three times as much page space as presenting it in tabular format. This usually occurs when four or more sets of data are to be presented.

However, thoughtful preparation makes the difference between a numerical table that confuses and one that informs the reader. Tables that communicate the quantitative aspects of data are effective only when the data are arranged so that their significance is obvious at a glance.

Understand how tables are constructed

In order to discuss table organization, it helps to know how table parts are named (Fig. 4.1). The column headings are known collectively as the *box heading*, and the group of row headings is called the *stub*. The *field* is the set of cells or spaces in the table's body that carries the numerical data, descriptive terms, or phrases which illustrate the message carried by the table. A *spanner* is a horizontal line used to indicate secondary column headings. A heading set above a spanner subsumes the subheads set under the spanner. Numbers in table columns are aligned on the decimal point. This is true even if the decimal point is implied rather than actually being included.

Understand basic printers' terms

In printing, a *point* is a unit measure for type, one point being approximately 1/72 of an inch. Historically, the point size of type was a measurement of the body on which the characters were set. The space between lines (called *leading*

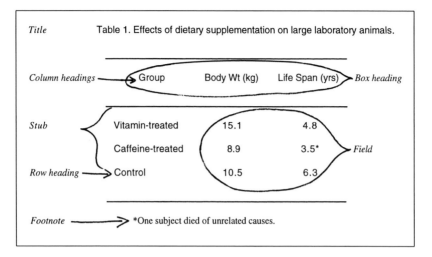

Fig. 4.1. Usual parts of a table and their names.

and pronounced "ledding") also was – and is – measured in points. For most typefaces, the size in points approximates the distance between the tops of the tallest letters (which may be either the capitals or the lowercase letters with ascenders, like *b* and *h*) and the bottoms of the letters with descenders, like *p* and *q*. The length of a line of type is measured in *picas*, one pica being equal to 12 points, or about 1/6 of an inch.

Because picas, used to measure a page of type, are not exactly compatible with inches, used to measure the size of a page after it has been trimmed, many manuscript editors use a pica rule (also called pica stick, line gauge, or publisher's type scale) to check page and type measurements. Such tools come in various designs (Fig. 4.2). One edge is always divided into picas and half-picas (i.e., 12- and 6-point divisions).

Use space efficiently

Experiment with table shapes. Provide enough spacing between rows and columns to create a perceptual order to the data, but do not space out columns artificially just to fill a page. It is easy to create too much vertical or horizontal emphasis when designing a table. To improve the table, adjust the space.

Most journals are printed in either a one-column or two-column format. Publications with a one-column format usually handle wide tables better than those with a two-column format; the latter will generally try to fit smaller tables into the width of a single column. Whenever possible, design tables (and figures, see below) to fit the width of a page or better yet, a column of text. In most scientific publications, narrow tables will stand a better chance of being printed close to the corresponding text.

To estimate how wide the table would be if set in type, count the number of

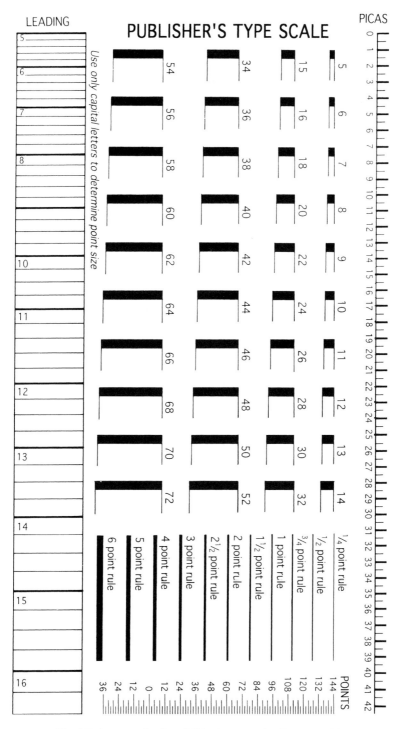

Fig. 4.2. An example of a publisher's type scale. Courtesy of Computer Support Corporation, Dallas, TX.

characters and spaces (allowing three between each pair of columns) in the longest line. If the count exceeds 50, the table is not likely to fit across the width of one column of a typical two-column format. If the count exceeds 100, the table will not fit across the width of most journal pages. However, because journal page sizes vary, check examples of single or double column tables in the targeted journal, and do not exceed the available character count.

If a table is too wide, delete a column, combine two or more columns, or rearrange the data, interchanging side headings (stub) and column headings (box) to form a vertical table. Reorienting the table is particularly desirable if the ratio of the number of column headings to the number of row headings is greater than 2:1. For example, a wide table such as Table 4.3 can be flipped efficiently to read like Table 4.4.

Other straightforward but often overlooked strategies for condensing tables include eliminating repeated words and economizing on heading lengths by judicious use of abbreviations. When all entries in a column or row are identical, omit that column or row. Note that result in the text, a table footnote, or table title.

The data may also be divided and presented in two or more smaller tables. Consider whether the material in a complex table really must be presented as one unit.

Table 4.3. *Wide table that would fit on a single-column page*

MAb	A5969	F	6/85	tS-11	R	S6	K503
	Assay scores (range 0–4) determined for various MG strains						
8F7/F	4	4	4	4	3	3	0
4G1/F	4	4	3	3	3	3	0

Table 4.4. *Modification of Table 4.3 to fit one side of a double-column layout*

MG strains	MAb 8F7/F	MAb 4G1/F
	Assay scores (range 0–4)	
A5969	4	4
F	4	4
6/85	4	3
tS-11	4	3
R	3	3
S6	3	3
K503	0	0

Draft concise table titles

Unlike figure legends, which are often listed together on a separate page from the text in a typescript, table titles are placed directly above each table. An effective table title should include not only the general subject ("Deer deaths in Wisconsin") but enough detail to make sense without the text ("Incidence of white-tailed deer fatalities in Wisconsin, 1995–2000").

Some journals allow or require brief descriptions of methods or experimental design to follow the title; others treat such information as a footnote below the table. In either case, keep them brief. They are generally printed in smaller text and when lengthy are difficult to read.

Help readers make comparisons by organizing tables logically

Remember, the reason for using tables is to help readers compare data, both within and between tables. Readers can compare items down a column more easily than across a row. Unless there is a valid reason to do otherwise, place independent variables in rows and dependent variables in columns. (Oversized tables can be an exception, see below.)

When the reader scans the column headings from left to right, and the stub headings from top to bottom, some sort of order should be apparent in both. Pre-treatment measurements, for example, might precede post-treatment ones; disease symptoms could be arranged from mildest to most severe. If there is no compelling reason for some other type of order, even listing material in rows or columns by the size of the numbers will help readers make mental comparisons.

The poorest sort of arrangement appears in analyses where data are arranged by arbitrary numbering of experimental subjects. Unless the numbers are truly relevant to understanding the results and some sort of explanatory code is included, experimental designations (A-307, D-10, and PC-2069) mean nothing to anyone but the investigator. In most cases, one can number the subjects by a conventional numeric system if they must be noted individually in the text. If they do not need individual mention in the text, omit subject numbers entirely in the accompanying table.

Research on illustration effectiveness (Macdonald-Ross, 1977a,b) suggests giving row and column averages as reference points. These averages can provide a visual focus that allows readers to inspect the data easily. However, do not clutter up a table with columns of numbers which could easily be derived from other columns by simple arithmetic.

To facilitate comparison between tables, be consistent in their presentation. Use the same terminology and similar titles and headings. Sometimes, as in many clinical papers, the title of the first table can be used to identify the main component of the results for the sequence of tables, with shorter titles for the tables that follow. For example, the first table in your review of 25 cases of puncture wounds might be titled "Puncture wounds of the canine abdomen: clinical features." The second table could be titled simply "Operative findings and postoperative course."

Avoid grossly oversized tables

Broadside tables – tables so wide that they must be printed at right angles to the text – are an inconvenience to readers who must turn the journal sideways to read them. Likewise, lengthy tables that spill over from one printed page to another are difficult for printers to align and difficult for readers to use. Some journals flatly refuse to print such tables. Double space everything in the table. If too long for a single sheet, continue on a second sheet, repeating all column and line headings. Absolutely no one is fooled by photocopied reductions or use of a smaller type font, techniques that simply annoy editors, reviewers, and typesetters, and may result in rejection of the typescript.

Large compilations of data often include information that is nonessential to the manuscript's purpose. Before altering the table's format, ask (1) whether all the information in the table actually is necessary, and (2) whether it must be presented in its current form. Does the reader need to know individual test results, or might summary statistics (such as mean, standard deviation, range, or median) be sufficient?

This is not the time to be sentimental. Numbers are not sacred simply because they have been collected, no matter how much work was involved in that collection. If you feel strongly that some readers of your condensed table will be vitally interested in more details long after you are able to provide them personally, consider placing your reams of data in permanent storage. The National Auxiliary Publications Service (NAPS) (Burrows Systems, 248 Hempstead Turnpike, West Hempstead, NY 11552) provides archiving. The editor of the journal in which reference to the deposited material will be made usually arranges for the deposit of such material. Detailed information on how to access this adjunct material must be clearly given in the acknowledgments section or as a footnote in a format suggested by NAPS.

Watch the details!

An effective table results from attention to a myriad of details. Study the format used by your journal. Consult *Instructions to Authors* and recent journal issues for table style, and mimic this style carefully. If the journal doesn't specify details of table style (and many do not), these details can usually be deduced from tables that have appeared in recent issues.

Note the style of table numbers and titles, box headings, subheadings, field entries, and footnotes. Check the use of horizontal and vertical rules. See where and how sample sizes ($n = 230$) are reported, and remember to include them. Without sample size information your study may have little worth to others.

For numerical data, use decimals rather than fractions to express parts of a whole number. Do not switch units of measure within a column. Instead, restructure the table so that the second kind of unit and accompanying data appear in another column. Likewise, do not mix units in a single column of data. Instead, change one of the units to an equivalent number of the other so that a single heading can apply to all.

Indicate units in column headings. If row headings designate numerical data, include the appropriate unit of measure immediately after or below the headings, either within parentheses or after a comma, depending on the journal's style.

Fill all cells in the field. This can be done in various ways. One system is to use ellipses (. . .) instead of dashes for a missing entry, *ND* for "not done," and *NA* for "not applicable" or "not available." For maximal clarity, some writers also append a footnote to the table to explain these abbreviations.

Symbols (*, #) or lowercase letters are usually used to indicate table footnotes. Numbers might be mistaken for data in a numerical table.

Unless otherwise specified, use Arabic numerals to sequentially identify each of your tables.

KNOW WHEN AND HOW TO INCLUDE FIGURES

In the parlance of the science editor, any visual aids that are not tables are figures. They may be numerically based (the many kinds of graphs), documentary (photographs, machine printouts), or explanatory (drawings, diagrams). Paradoxically, while figures themselves are often overused, many types are underutilized. The checklist that began this chapter (Table 4.1) should help expand your list of possibilities. For additional ideas, see Briscoe (1996), Brock (1990), and Simmonds and Reynolds (1994).

Before considering each of these basic figure types in turn, allow us to offer some suggestions that apply to them all.

Decide when a figure is appropriate

Figures should be included in a scientific paper when they are needed for evidence, efficiency, or emphasis. Evidence is easy. If something of vital interest occurs during a clinical trial or a case study, one naturally wants to document it with a photograph. During a taxonomic study, an unusual structure or notable range in a character's expression seems to beg for illustration.

Efficiency implies that the figure is the most succinct and effective way to make a particular point. When appropriate, combine material. Draw several curves on a single graph. Combine diagrams to illustrate steps in a procedure. Illustrations well prepared for an oral presentation generally present a relatively limited amount of information; they usually can and should be combined for publication.

Emphasis is a major reason for using illustrations in a spoken talk. However, it is not a sufficient reason for including figures in a published paper. Never include figures just because they happen to be available. Most editors will stringently assess each figure's usefulness in communicating the message of the paper.

Make figures both independent and indispensable

A figure and its legend should be a complete unit of communication, just like a table with its accompanying material. All symbols and images within the figure should be explained. If necessary for understanding, experimental details should be given in the legend about how the figure was obtained. If appropriate, matters such as degree of magnification and type of stain should be included. Do not take chances on losing readers to frustration. During the editing stages, show your illustrations to someone who knows little or nothing about your research. Then listen, and be prepared to address the sometimes surprising questions your illustrations will raise.

While visual aids must be independent of the text, they also must be indispensable to its story. As Bjelland (1990, p. 79) says, "Visuals must mesh with your text, like two gears that drive a machine. They must work in concert, each dependent on the other, to describe an object, a process, or a concept." Readers almost always look at illustrative material first. Good visual materials should spark reader interest, and interested readers will have questions. To be effective, use the text to answer these questions.

Prepare attractive figures, but beware of "glitziness"

Even a cursory look through the scientific literature will reveal that published illustrations differ widely in their quality. Many details in format lettering and labeling call for careful attention, and seemingly small things can make the difference between a so-so illustration and an excellent one. For example, lines should not be less than 0.4 mm thick and symbols not less than 2.5 mm in diameter on original artwork. If professional graphic artists and photographers are available, consult them, and provide them with samples from the journal.

Increasingly, scientists are using their computers (with associated peripherals such as scanners and laser printers) to prepare their graphic illustrations. If you decide to prepare the illustrations yourself, investigate the latest software and printer requirements and learn how to use them.

Finally, watch out for what Peterson (1993) calls "glitziness." It is easy to become caught up in the capabilities of sophisticated graphics software capabilities. Some truly beautiful illustrations are possible. However, be aware that they can present a new set of communication pitfalls. Even when there is no overt attempt to deceive, it is possible to present a compelling visualization which through choice of perspective can obscure or distort data.

Pay attention to size and scale

Reducing the size of artwork for publication can do strange things to scale. Reduction minimizes some flaws, but accentuates others. Use a reduction wheel, hand-held reducing lens, or a photocopier with reduction abilities to check what a figure will look like after reduction.

A horizontal rectangle, with a longer horizontal than vertical axis, will usually fit within the layout of a journal's page. (A ratio of 2 vertical units to 3 horizontal units is considered especially pleasing.) Vertical rectangles often need reduction; whenever possible, reformat them to a square or horizontal rectangle.

After reduction of the illustration for publication, the capital letters in written material on the figure should be about 2.0 mm in height. Lines for the x- and y-axes and trend lines in graphs should be no wider than the width of the lines making up the letters. Points on curves in graphs should not be so large as to merge upon reduction.

If the size of the subject of a photograph is important, include a short scale line to indicate dimensions. If possible, lay a centimeter–millimeter rule in the field so that it will be visible in the finished photograph. Apply a scale to a photomicrograph.

Write and position legends carefully

Legends (explanatory titles or captions) are a vital part of every figure, not a tacked-on afterthought. When readers turn a page, they look first at illustrations, then at the legends. Each title should orient the readers toward the figure's meaning and enable them to identify its components without referring to the text. It should also differentiate that particular figure from all other illustrations in the paper.

Like a table title, a figure legend should be brief – 8 to 12 words, as a rule of thumb – and need not be a complete sentence. However, a good legend should contain enough detail for readers to understand the illustration. A legend such as "Fig. 1. Graph of relevant data" is too vague. Alternatively, "Fig. 1. Outcome of multifactorial analysis of relationship between symptoms, chronology of appearance, diagnostic signs, blood work constants from the literature, health outcome, and other parameters for selected group of 15 adult ostriches" is so over-specified that it buries the identity of the figure and exhausts the reader. Strike a middle ground – "Fig. 1. Multifactorial analysis of health records of 15 adult ostriches" – and assign the rest of the information to the text.

In the final version of the typescript, figure legends should be listed (double spaced) on a sheet of paper separate from the text, usually appended to the end of the typescript. When prepared for a verbal presentation as a slide or transparency, however, figures should have the legend placed directly on them.

USE GRAPHS TO PROMOTE UNDERSTANDING OF NUMERICAL RESULTS

Tables present results; graphs promote understanding of results and suggest interpretations of their meaning and relationships. Most graphs are based on a set of numbers, just as most tables are. But because graphs are fundamentally pictures rather than a set of numbers, information generally is easier for the reader to grasp than if it were printed in columns.

Consider graphing data when you feel that the relationships are more vital to your message than the actual numerical values themselves. Thus, you might use a graph to present trends dealing with two related variables, one or more variables changing through time, or data interesting for the magnitudes of differences which might be related to unknown factors or experimental manipulations.

A graph always shows how one parameter varies relative to changes in another. One factor may be controlled and varied (temperature, for example) while some effect of this change is measured. Alternatively, the effect of changes in some uncontrollable factor such as time may be measured. Temperature and time in these examples are independent variables, which are usually plotted in relation to the horizontal (x) axis. The effect these changes have on something else (the dependent variable) is normally plotted in relation to the vertical (y) axis.

A range of computer programs can produce sophisticated graphs with the touch of a finger. Use them initially to construct various graphic presentations of the data and consider the alternatives. Then modify such aspects as fonts, type size, shadings, and symbols to produce visually dynamic illustrations. Remember, however, that legibility and comprehensibility should remain the most important criteria. Common errors in graphical data are discussed by Cleveland (1994).

Keep line graphs simple

Line graphs (Fig. 4.3) visually show continuous variables such as movements over time. They range from straightforward visual representations of trends to depictions of complex advanced statistical analyses.

Line graphs are probably the most popular of all graph styles in scientific writing. Unfortunately, studies have shown that many readers lack the skills to interpret them (Macdonald-Ross, 1977a). If you decide to use line graphs, keep

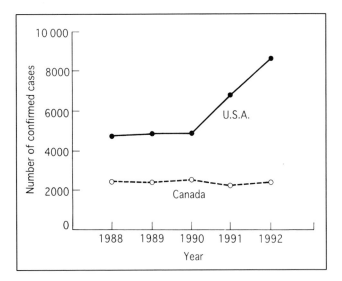

Fig. 4.3. This effective line graph shows changes in rabies disease incidence over time.

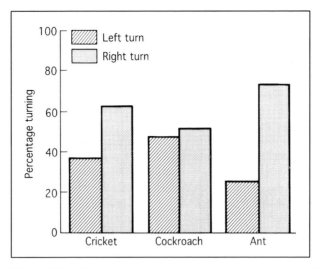

Fig. 4.4. This effective bar graph relates insect type to turning choices.

them as simple as possible. Visually distinguish different lines by using different symbols, and label each line carefully.

Limit logarithmic and scatter graphs to professional audiences

A logarithmic graph has a series of open and grouped vertical lines in which the top and bottom of each group, called a cycle, is a decimal or multiple of ten. It is commonly but not exclusively used to compare data in which rate of change is more important than quantity of change. (An exception sometimes encountered in medical writing is the dose-response curve. Dose is logarithmically related to response in terms of number of receptors stimulated.) A logarithmic graph also is frequently used when the vertical range is so large that it is difficult to fit on a normal graph. However, because nonscientific readers may not be familiar with a logarithmic scale, they can find such graphs confusing.

Scatter graphs, which sometimes are charted logarithmically, use single unconnected dots to plot instances where two variables (one on each axis) meet. The pattern of the dots expresses the relationship (a diagonal trend, which is sometimes approximated by a line on the chart) or lack of a relationship (random scatter) between the variables. Interpreting scatter graphs also can be difficult for nonscientific readers.

If you choose to use either of these graphing techniques, it is imperative that their significance be explained and discussed clearly in the text.

Reveal general relationships with bar graphs

Bar graphs (Fig. 4.4) (also sometimes called column graphs) are used to present discrete variables in a visually forceful way. They are a single axis graph used to compare size and magnitude of discontinuous data. They are superior to circle and line graphs for showing relationships, magnitudes, and distributions (Macdonald-Ross, 1977b). On the negative side, bar graphs generally provide a relatively small amount of information while taking up a fairly large amount of space.

The bars may run either vertically or horizontally, but are most effective when they run in the direction in which people expect to see them. Thus, vertical bars are usually used for such data as temperature and weight, horizontal bars for distance, time, and speed. Whatever type of bar graph you choose, make the bars the same width, and the space between bars or bar groups one-half of a bar width.

Subdividing bars by shading or cross-hatching adds another dimension of information. Divided bar graphs, for example, can compare percentages of a whole rather than relative size. In this, they function much like pie charts but are less effective. Superficially similar to bar graphs, histograms are two axis graphs that typically show frequency distributions by use of a series of contiguous rectangular bars.

Illustrate the relationship of parts to a whole with divided-circle graphs

Most of the time, bar graphs seem to be superior to circle and line graphs for presenting information. However, divided-circle graphs (Fig. 4.5), also called pie charts, are well suited for showing the relationship of a number of parts to the whole.

Although pie charts make a striking visual display, they present a fundamental problem – the impossibility of comparing areas. They are generally used best as attention-getting devices, and even then, only when comparing five or fewer

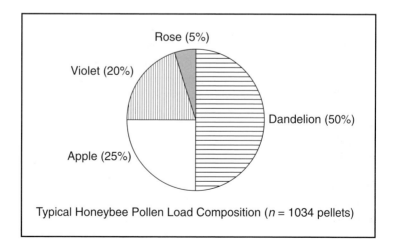

Fig. 4.5. This effective divided-circle graph shows which flowers contribute to a typical honeybee pollen load. To help readers compare the proportions, percentages are included.

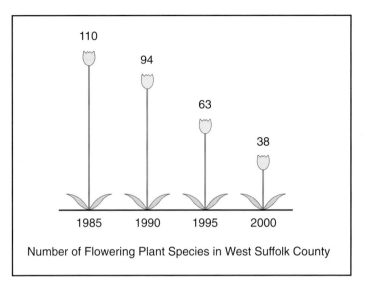

Fig. 4.6. In this effective pictograph, the length of the flower stems corresponds to the number of plant species.

items. Pie charts are most effective when the segments are arranged by size, with the largest slice beginning at twelve o'clock. Continue placing progressively smaller segments clockwise. Note that some graphics software programs generate counterclockwise charts. Include no slices smaller than about 5% (18 degrees).

Let pictographs show numerical relationships in a visually symbolic manner

Pictographs are essentially bar graphs composed of pictures. They can be very visually effective.

Pictographs are of two basic types. In one, each symbol corresponds to a total quantity (Fig. 4.6). In the other, uniformly sized symbols each represent a unit amount with a key provided that explains their meaning (Fig. 4.7). Often the

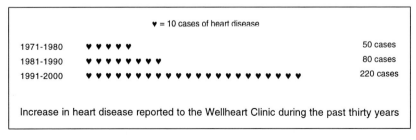

Fig. 4.7. A pictograph that uses heart symbols to show disease incidence effectively reflects the subject of the graph.

precise actual numbers are posted at the end of each row or column, since such graphs present an approximation.

Perhaps because their construction historically has fallen within the domain of graphic artists, pictographs rarely appear in scientific writing, though they might provide welcome variety. With the ease with which they can be constructed using computer graphics software and clip art, they deserve wider use. They are especially appropriate and effective for illustrating oral and poster presentations. If you choose to use this type of illustration, remember that pictographs are most effective when the symbols chosen represent the subject matter and are arranged in a way that presents an organized message.

Keep graphs visually honest

Graphs can be distorted in many ways, from finagling line fits to deleting data points that do not fit the curve to making data points so large that almost any curve would pass through them. A graph is dishonest if it leads readers to come away with a disproportionate sense of the relationship it portrays.

While you certainly want to make readers aware of certain trends, as a scientist, you have the responsibility not to distort the importance of any trend, tempting as this may be. There are no iron-clad procedures to guarantee that your illustrations will accent trends without distorting them, but here are a few suggestions.

Begin at zero for the scales used for the axes of a graph whenever possible; choose these scales carefully and mark them clearly. Sometimes a valid trend would disappear on a scale with a zero axis, and all the data points would bunch up at the top. In this case, signal readers that the graph's axis is not at zero, either with a statement in the text or with a break in the axis.

If a point represents the mean of a number of observations, indicate the magnitude of the variability by a vertical line centered at each point. State whether standard error (SE) or standard deviation (SD) is used and specify number of observations or sample sizes.

When two or more graphs or other figures are to be compared, draw them to the same scale. If possible, place them side by side. If you juxtapose graphs with different scales, readers may mistakenly assume that the scales are the same.

Remember the limitations of your data. The extrapolation of a line or a curve beyond the points shown on a graph may mislead both the writer and the reader. As Winston Churchill is said to have remarked in another context, "It is wise to look ahead but foolish to look further than you can see."

Line graphs need special attention. A false impression may be given if successive discontinuous data points on a graph are connected. It is better to present such information as a bar graph or to leave the points on the graph without connecting lines.

USE DOCUMENTARY ILLUSTRATIONS EFFECTIVELY

A second category of visual aids includes those image-based illustrations that document discoveries. This is the category most people think of when they hear that a paper has "figures." The photograph of a new organism, the tracing from an oscillograph, the radiographic image of a patient's bone deformity . . . all would belong here, and all would be submitted as a photographic copy. (Remember, an astute scientific writer rarely submits the original image, and never sends the sole copy of anything!)

When it comes to showing exactly what something looks like, nothing beats the realism of a photograph. A photograph carries a great deal of credibility; the reader knows that the object being photographed really exists. It also usually costs less to produce than a diagram or line drawing.

At the same time, the realism of a photograph can be disadvantageous. It may include clutter, extraneous information, or components you would rather not show. It will usually only show surfaces, not the components or interior parts that a line drawing or diagrammatic exploded view can provide. Furthermore, obtaining a photograph of high enough quality to merit publication can be difficult under some circumstances, such as during biological field work. Sometimes a traditional drawing is a better choice.

Obtain the best documentation possible

When photographs seem called for, take a number of shots, both in color and in black and white using a range of exposures. Focus sharply. Provide a plain, uncluttered background that does not draw attention away from the object you're depicting. Be alert to the distracting presence of miscellaneous items, such as soft drink cans. Try a variety of angles, and take more than one photograph at each exposure setting. Taking extra exposures at the time of photography is better than making copies later. Duplicating transparencies and negatives from their originals usually leads to degrading of color quality and image sharpness.

Use both color and monochrome film for the original photographs. Colored pictures usually are preferred for oral or poster presentations, whereas most journal photographs are black and white images. Black and white prints can made from color transparencies or color prints, but are never quite as good as photographs made directly in black and white. Use of digital cameras alleviates this concern since their images can be made into either type of print.

Sometimes, color illustration is necessary for reasons of evidence, efficiency, or emphasis. For example, color could be vital in illustrations of faint rashes, subtle histologic stain colors, or multicolor scan images. Be sure to investigate the journal's policy on – and charges for – use of color; few journals will publish color illustrations without passing the cost on to the author. Note also that journals generally prefer color transparencies (slides) and color negatives (negatives for color prints) to color prints.

Compose the illustration to help the reader

After a photograph has passed the tests of quality and message, it should be tailored to give the reader as much help as possible. Crop the print to a shape suitable for the journal without reduction in size. Select the center of the field to coincide with the center of interest. Affix letters and arrows identifying features of interest. Keep any lettering horizontal and of an appropriately consistent size and contrast for easy reading. Include in the legend a key to any symbols used. If appropriate, in the corner of the photograph include a bar to represent a length appropriate to the scale. Finally, consider grouping related figures into a single plate to fill an entire printed page in the final publication.

USE EXPLANATORY ARTWORK EFFECTIVELY

The third category of figures are those produced to communicate organization, illustrate basic principles, or otherwise explain text materials. It includes all of those flow charts, diagrams, gazintas, maps, algorithms, and line art which some people characterize as "illustrations" as opposed to tables and photographs.

The effectiveness of explanatory artwork depends upon how well it focuses audience attention. This type of artwork must show the specific details of key features while omitting the distraction caused by extraneous details. A common mistake is to present a figure that is much more complex than the accompanying prose. Such illustrations confuse rather than inform readers.

What is a gazinta?

Science writer Harley Bjelland (1990, p. 83) uses the term *gazinta*, derived from the expression "goes into," to encompass those visuals that show the hierarchy and complexity of actions within an object, idea, or organization. A gazinta shows organization and interaction.

One type of gazinta, the drawing tree (Fig. 4.8), is essentially static. It shows the subassemblies that make up an assembly and the assemblies that make up an object or an organization. In a drawing tree, all subassemblies of the same relative importance or size appear on the same vertical level. As you progress from the bottom to the top of the tree, the subassemblies become larger, more complex, and fewer in number.

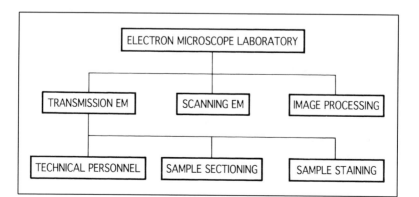

Fig. 4.8. A typical drawing tree gazinta describes a relatively stable situation.

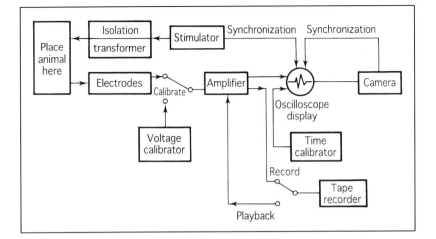

Fig. 4.9. A typical block diagram gazinta depicts a procedure. (Redrawn after Rogoff, J. B. and S. Reiner, 1961.)

The other main type of gazinta, the block diagram (Fig. 4.9), depicts objects or materials in action. The block diagram is one of the most often used visuals in engineering and science to show how things interact with each other, be they electrical, mechanical, chemical, biological, or some combination of these.

Bjelland (1990) considers block diagrams to be the most useful visual aids for any type of technical writing, and recommends these guidelines. To reduce confusion, show only major actions and interactions, and limit the number of blocks to no more than 8 to 10. Use short functional names for each block, and use exactly the same name in the accompanying text. Keep the functional level the same within a specific block diagram. If abbreviations or specialized terms are used in the diagram, define them the first time they appear in the accompanying text or include them in the legend.

Indicate each flow with a different type of coded line, reserving solid lines for the primary flow. Use arrowheads to indicate direction, which should flow the way one would read standard printed information. In the text, use an order of presentation that follows the direction of flow on the diagram and that carries the flow through the entire diagram.

Guide readers through sequential processes with algorithms

An algorithm (Fig. 4.10) is a special method of solving a certain kind of problem. It has been defined as "a means of reaching a decision by considering only those factors which are relevant to that particular decision" (Wheatley and Unwin, 1972, p. 10). Algorithms include such varied items as decision charts, decision tables, flowcharts, tree diagrams, taxonomic keys, and income tax forms. What they have in common is a way of guiding the reader through a series of steps in a sequential manner.

Algorithms have an important place in technical communication, and deserve to be more widely used. Once people become familiar with their use,

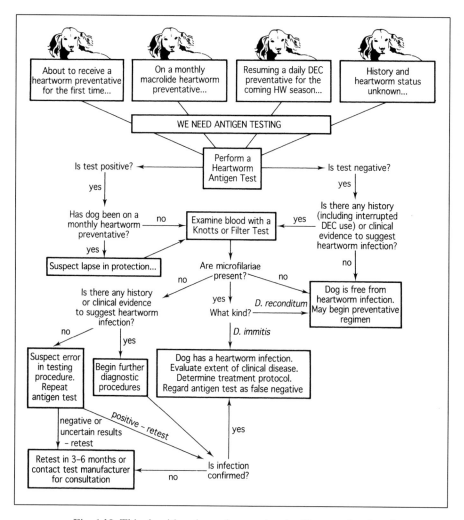

Fig. 4.10. This algorithm shows the steps involved in screening dogs for canine heartworm infection.

they generally find algorithms quicker and easier to follow than narrative instructions.

If you have occasion to use algorithms, study their use in your respective discipline, and follow style guidelines. Remember that their strength lies in their clarity, so they must be kept uncrowded and free of extraneous detail.

Use traditional drawings to focus on essentials

Not surprisingly, pen-and-ink artwork has long been an integral part of technical communication, particularly in the biological and medical sciences. If

Exercise 4–1. Table and figure format choices

The choice of a format in which to present data is a judgment call. What would you use for the examples below? Your choices need not match ours if you feel you have sound justification for them.

1. You've gathered a series of data concerning serum electrolyte values and acid–base variables for patients with Rocky Mountain spotted fever. How should you present this information?

2. You've examined mortality rates for male and female cats with thyroid disease in individual states of the United States. Should you use a table, graph, or figure?

3. You've measured maximum systolic blood pressure after giving white rats various doses of epinephrine, and have measured changes in their blood pressure throughout a 2-week period. You also have a really nice photograph of one of your control rats. What should you publish, and in what form?

4. In a case series study, you have collected data from a physical examination of animals at admittance, from observations during the course of the illness, and from final autopsies. You've decided to present the data in a table; how should they be arranged?

5. You have written a paper about a new species of a bacterial pathogen implicated in a case of pneumonia. You have a chest roentgenogram showing typical findings of pneumonia, and an electronmicrograph of newly discovered structural details of the bacterium's flagellum. Should you include either or both in your paper?

6. You have identified a genetic syndrome that appears in members of a plant lineage as a Mendelian autosomal dominant trait. Should you present your evidence as a table, a graph, or text?

7. You have researched deaths from mycoplasmal diseases in turkeys and ducks, and found a significant difference in mortality rates. How should you show this difference?

carefully prepared, two- or three-dimensional renderings of an object are often clearer than a photograph, and preferable to it. The major advantage of drawings is that you can control the amount of precision, deleting extraneous details. Drawings also permit unique perspectives such as cutaway, blow-up, and exploded views.

Dozens of computer graphics packages are on the market. Some are very good, but there is a vast difference between creating artwork on a computer and creating it with pen and ink on paper. For some people, producing their own drawings is exhilarating. If you are not one of them, employ a graphic designer or professional artist. For best results, communicate carefully and allow sufficient lead time for the project. Remember that artists aren't technical experts. Sketch your ideas, explain your terms, provide correct spellings, and check everything carefully for errors during preparation of the artwork.

5

Revising structure and style

> On the whole, I think the pain which my father took over the literary part of the work was very remarkable. He often laughed or grumbled at himself for the difficulty which he found in writing English, saying, for instance, that if a bad arrangement of a sentence was possible, he would be sure to adopt it .... When a sentence got hopelessly involved, he would ask himself "now what do you want to say?" and his answer written down, would often disentangle the confusion.
>
> *Charles Darwin's son, Francis*

To see how difficult writing is, even for experienced writers, we have only to study their manuscripts: They are full of alterations, crossings out, additions, loops, arrows, blots. The apparent spontaneity of easy-reading prose is the result of hard work.

Those who can write a finished document and first draft at the same time are few, and might be compared to the rare musical prodigy who can play symphonies without ever taking a music lesson. Revision most often is the step in scientific writing that separates the beginner from the master craftsman. It's the reason why professional writers have such big wastebaskets! They keep working on a piece until it is right.

Two processes are involved in written communication. The first, in your mind, is the selection of words to express your thoughts. The second, in the mind of the reader, is the conversion of the written words into thoughts. The essential difficulty is in trying to ensure that the thoughts created in the mind of the reader are the same thoughts that were in your mind. Revisions are just a way to fine-tune this transfer.

The word "revise" comes from the Latin, *revidere* – to see again. It means a willingness to make changes, often big changes. It's no accident that a synonym for "first draft" is "rough draft." Most are disjointed and overwritten. They contain grammatical errors, jargon, contractions, wordiness, repetition . . . and this is fine! We write as we speak. However, there are many differences between spoken language and written language. In spoken language, phrases and ideas are often repeated, in order to give a listener additional clues to the message. In written language, a reader can, if necessary, reread a passage. The inflection and timing clues are absent. Meaning depends entirely on word choice. Revision of the conversational-style first draft, therefore, is essential if you want to come up with a well-written scientific paper.

Remember the Process Approach we introduced back in Chapter 1? It involved methodically breaking the writing task into discrete stages (see Table 1.3), and tackling each one systematically, efficiently, and effectively. Revising by this approach entails a series of nested steps, each concentrating on successively finer points. The first revision concentrates on the document's structure and basic style, examining both brevity and clarity. That step is the focus of this chapter.

Style-polishing may have been what you have been expecting – and dreading – from the start. This stage of writing well can be hard work, but stick with us. Mastering the fundamentals of scientific style demands no special inspiration or genius that stamps a person as different from all others. It is simply a skill akin to doing crossword puzzles or solving logic puzzles. It is a word game, itself, in which the winning combination is a sort of functional beauty that arises from barrier-free communication.

Don't get so close to the supposed difficulties that you lose sight of the pleasure in it. There is pleasure to be derived from any effort of creative activity, including this one. Like the hand-turned table you might build or the picture you might paint, each article you write is an original vehicle of self-expression. Your information and ideas will be expressed in a way which is your own. The material you choose to include, the arrangement of your arguments, the criticisms you raise, and the conclusions you reach, all reflect your own personality and intellect.

Let's not be afraid also to acknowledge that pleasure comes from writing something which will affect other people. Part of the enjoyment of writing well is that of meeting the challenge of doing your best to present information and ideas directly and forcefully, to help the reader along, and to affect the reader in a chosen way.

STRUCTURAL CHANGES COME FIRST

Begin with the big picture: basic organization and logic. Start with a complete rereading of the rough draft. Viewing paper copy is particularly important if you have been using word processing. The computer screen shows only a small part of the typescript at a time. Some problems – such as scrambled organization, or redundancy – simply aren't very noticeable unless several pages of the typescript are spread out in front of you.

Make two or more paper copies of the document. If your first draft has been typed or written by hand, run it through a photocopy machine. If it has been word processed, print it in duplicate. Read one copy. Write notes in its margins such as "delete," "move to discussion," or "combine Tables 1 and 2." Later you will follow the notes on the first copy as you physically cut up the second copy and tape parts together in the new order. Save this annotated copy as a safeguard against accidentally losing one or more paragraphs of text during your cut-and-paste work.

As you read the first draft, examine the order of presentation. Check whether all of your lines of reasoning hold up. Correct any misquotations. Evaluate your

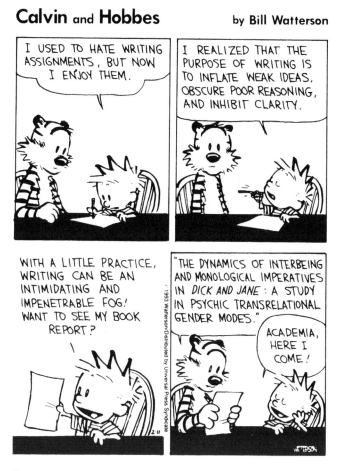

CALVIN AND HOBBES © 1993 Watterson. Reprinted with permission of
UNIVERSAL PRESS SYNDICATE. All rights reserved.

inclusion of literature citations. (A common tendency is to include references
that merely relate to the same complex of ideas, rather than having a true bearing
on the argument.) Combine or simplify tables where necessary. In short, do any
and all of your major cut-and-paste work.

Nine basic organizational questions need to be addressed in nearly every
paper. If any of them cause problems, refer to the material in Chapters 1 and 3.

Is the title accurate, succinct, and effective?

Titles are more effective when they begin with a keyword (see pages 68–69).
Check *Instructions to Authors* for any limits on title length. Subtitles, if allowed
and used, should be able to stand alone. They should not duplicate the main
title. Assure that the title is grammatically correct, and pay particular attention

to the placement of modifiers. Double meanings that arise from a misplaced or dangling modifier can quickly land you a spot in the Blooper Hall of Fame! (See pages 124–127 for more on this topic.)

Does the abstract represent all the content within the allowed length?

An abstract of a research report should include the study design, experimental subjects, methods, results, and interpretations. An abstract of a case report should briefly characterize the patient as well as the unusual features of the case. A review article abstract usually tells what the review is about, rather than representing its content in highly condensed form. (See pages 67–68.)

Does the introductory material set the stage adequately but concisely?

Remember the three-part format: orient the reader, disclose the gap to be filled, and present the question you propose to answer. At the end of the Introduction section, have you clearly spelled out the focus of your research? (See page 64.)

Is the rest of the text in the right sequence?

Most full-length research papers in scientific journals have a fairly conventional format, although the position of the abstract, acknowledgments, and footnoted material often varies. Case reports, review articles, editorials, and book reviews appear in many different formats, and are more likely to show deviations in sequence.

Is all of the text really needed?

Most first drafts are overwritten. Introductions explain more than most readers need to know. Results sections present data that have little or nothing to do with the main message of the paper. Discussions open with a statement of points made in the introduction, or run on with speculations about a study's findings that go far beyond hypotheses that could be tested in the near future.

Can some of the first draft be discarded? Does any of the text repeat information presented elsewhere in the document? It can be difficult to be as ruthless as necessary. You may be reluctant to leave out any text when you worked so hard getting it into the first draft. Remember that your document will be judged by content, not number of words. Readers will thank you only for a paper that gets to the point, sticks to it, and presents content directly relevant to that point.

Is any needed content missing?

Sometimes – especially if a writer is interrupted while working on the first draft – important material gets left out. Keep this question in mind, and such gaps will probably jump to your attention when you read through the first draft.

Do data in the text agree with data in the tables?

If you wrote the first draft with the tables before you, as we suggested, you should have no problems with this, but check anyway. Surprising things sometimes happen.

Are the correct references included?

Look for essential references that may be missing, and for references that are unnecessary. Repeat this step at the end of the revision process. The further along a typescript goes in the sequence of drafts, the more likely it is that changes have led to errors.

Use only the references needed to support key statements in the text. For example, if you must refer to a description of a disease so that you do not have to describe the disease, refer to one or two complete and reliable sources. Do not give an additional four or five or more to show that you are familiar with all of the related literature. For any methods previously described, direct the reader to relevant references, and include only enough detail to orient readers and alert them to any modifications you may have made.

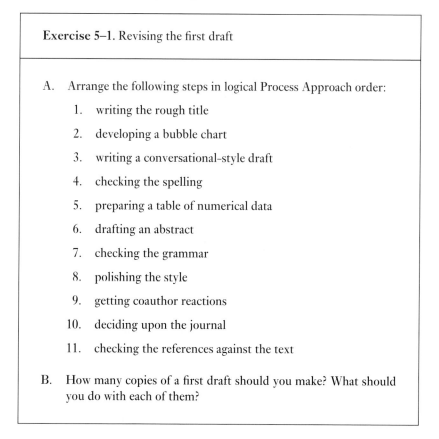

Exercise 5–1. Revising the first draft

A.   Arrange the following steps in logical Process Approach order:

1. writing the rough title

2. developing a bubble chart

3. writing a conversational-style draft

4. checking the spelling

5. preparing a table of numerical data

6. drafting an abstract

7. checking the grammar

8. polishing the style

9. getting coauthor reactions

10. deciding upon the journal

11. checking the references against the text

B.   How many copies of a first draft should you make? What should you do with each of them?

Theses and dissertations are sometimes an exception to this rule. Advisory committees may require extensive review and referencing to showcase a graduate student's mastery of the literature in a research field. Before the research papers that arise from this work are submitted for publication, however, remove all but the most directly relevant material.

Should any of the tables or illustrations be omitted? Restructured? Combined?

This is even more difficult to do than discarding text. If you followed the recommendations mentioned earlier, you have so far prepared only rough copies of tables and illustrations. Often at this stage, you'll find that tables can be rearranged or combined in ways that didn't occur to you when you began. If some of the data you collected are of only tangential importance to the basic research questions being addressed, delete them. There is no justification for including data simply on the grounds that you collected them, and someday you think someone somewhere might wish to know of them.

REVISE FOR CLARITY

A tongue-in-cheek key to understanding scientific writing

What the scientist said	What he meant
It has long been known that . . .	I haven't bothered to look up the original reference, but . . .
Of great theoretical and practical importance . . .	Interesting to me . . .
Typical results are shown . . .	The best results are shown . . .
It is suggested that; It is believed that; It may be that . . .	I think . . .
It is generally believed that . . .	A couple of other guys think so, too.
It is clear that much additional work will be required before a complete understanding . . .	I don't understand it.
Unfortunately, a quantitative theory to account for these results has not been formulated.	I can't think of one, and neither can anyone else.
Correct within an order of magnitude	Wrong.
Thanks are due to Joe Clotz for assistance with the experiments and to Boyton Fird for valuable discussion.	Clotz did the work, and Fird interpreted the data.

Author unknown

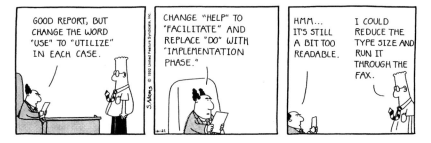

DILBERT © United Features Syndicate.

The simplest writing style is usually best. This does not mean that one should avoid technical words. They often are not only necessary, but the very best way to express a thought. It does mean that verbose words and phrases should not be included in a vain attempt to impress the reader with the writer's intellect and scientific status. Sentence structure should not have to be puzzled over. Paragraphs should not ramble on and on.

Clarity includes what some call "grace of expression." People have grace when they go beyond politeness and act with an eye to the needs and comfort of others. Graceful prose is much the same. It does not offend readers or divert their minds from the message. It does not try to impress readers with its erudition, or force them into side issues. It serves readers without imposing upon them. "Good prose is like a window pane," wrote George Orwell, the English essayist – it is transparent in the sense that it puts no visible obstacle between the reader and the message.

Although the content of a document is more likely to determine whether it is accepted for publication than is its prose style, gracefully written text gives readers a sense that the author has mastered his or her subject. The first of those readers will be the editor and the document reviewers.

Consider person and point of view

As a writer, you can choose to present a subject in a personal or impersonal manner. In a personal point of view, you play the role of writer and reporter openly, using *I, me,* and *my,* or *we, us,* and *our.* The impersonal point of view, on the other hand, requires avoiding all explicit reference to yourself.

As a writer, you also choose the level of formality of the writing, a closely related but independent factor. The decision is not solely between personal informality and impersonal formality; a personal point of view can accompany a very formal writing style.

On many occasions one point of view or the other is preferable. This book includes both. When we have offered you tips and suggestions, we've taken an openly personal point of view, feeling that it is a friendly approach to a very personal subject – your efforts at scientific writing. When we have had to present stern pronouncements or inflexible dictums, a more impersonal and formal style has often been used.

In their professional publications, scientists almost always maintain an impersonal writing style, which the scientific culture generally views as somehow having more prestige and objectivity. Usually, it is coupled with passive constructions (see pages 120–121) and avoidance of the first person.

Total avoidance of the first person in scientific text is neither necessary nor desirable, however, as increasing numbers of journal editors are realizing. It has been rumored that some journals do not allow the use of personal pronouns, but our informal survey of over 200 of them located none that formally specified this in their *Instructions to Authors*. We suspect that scientific writing's heavy reliance on the passive voice is more a matter of tradition than a formal requirement.

Using the first person is often shorter, simpler, and less pompous than avoiding it. For example, "the authors are prepared to argue" can be shortened to "we contend." "The authors wish to thank" can be shortened to "we thank." An added benefit is that active verb forms can replace passive ones, making it difficult to construct dangling participles.

When referring to published results and then giving one's own, directly claim the latter. A common source of confusion is narratives such as the one below. Whose results are whose? And who found which inconsistencies? Phrases such as "it was found that" leave readers wondering who made the discovery. They are best avoided.

> *Confusing:* This result was elucidated by Smith (1990) and Jones (1991). In these studies the authors found inconsistencies in the results. It was found that the data differed slightly.
>
> *Better:* Smith (1990) was first to explain this result; Jones (1991) expanded upon the idea. Our research uncovered minor inconsistencies in the data given in both of their studies.

When using the first person, employ it consistently and correctly. Sudden and illogical shifts in point of view make a document difficult to read.

> *Inconsistent:* We have reached the point where one should do further experiments. *[Does this mean we intend to do them? Or are we suggesting someone else should do it?]*
>
> *Better:* We have reached the point where we should do further experiments.
>
> *Unclear:* The authors established the gene-splicing service in 1976, and we have expanded it ever since. *[Are we and the authors one and the same?]*
>
> *Better:* We established the gene-splicing service in 1976 and have expanded it ever since.

One further point on correct use of the first person: When you are the sole author, do not refer to yourself as *we*. You must use *I* – unless you are a monarch or pregnant!

Exercise 5–2. Person and point of view

Change the use of third and first person in the following sentences. Many variations are possible.

1. The laboratory technician will find that the new procedure is an improvement; you will not need to sterilize the skin.

2. van Niel and colleagues showed that some bacteria do not give off molecular oxygen but the authors herein contend that they still photosynthesize.

3. The authors wish to gratefully acknowledge and thank Dr C. F. Snow for technical assistance and expertise.

4. It was found that the disease is contagious and that you should avoid contamination (van der Veen, 1850); the author concurs that cleanliness is essential.

5. It is postulated by the author, working alone and writing herein, that we have discovered a new species of *Australopithecus*.

Pay attention to factors that influence readability

One of the most common complaints about scientific documents is that they difficult to read because of the ponderous complexity and length of their words, sentences, and paragraphs. To present ideas effectively, minimize the combined weight of these factors. As the complexity and length of words increase, the complexity and length of sentences and paragraphs should be reduced to compensate.

To reading experts, the term "readability" refers to aspects of writing that can be measured and subjected to a formula. Readability formulas such as Fry, Flesch, Fog, and Kincaid are based on the relationships between average word length (or number of syllables) and average sentence length. Various ratios between the two allow a document's readability to be ranked by difficulty or by grade. Readability formulas are frequently used, partly because they are widely available on computer software.

Scores obtained with these formulas can be helpful in tailoring material to a particular audience, or in maintaining some uniformity in multiauthored compilations. However, they do not adequately address many important elements of scientific writing. Difficulty of content is ignored, as is the recognition factor. Some multisyllable medical terms are easily and immediately recognized, even by general readers. Conversely, highly technical material may use very short words and be easy to read, but still be difficult for any but a few specialists to comprehend. Finally, even such a simple matter as document design can affect readability.

Strive for sentences of about 20 words

For maximal readability, most sentences in most scientific prose should be about 15 to 20 words long. This is an easy matter to determine with a word processing program. Sentences with more than 40 words generally are too long. If sentences consistently include fewer than 12 words – a rare situation in scientific writing – consider linking and expanding some of them. Usually, a set of sentences 15–20 words long will express an idea in somewhat fewer words than a set of overly long or short sentences does.

> *Too long:* Two canine cadavers with orthopedic abnormalities were identified which included a first dog that had an unusual deformity secondary to premature closure of the distal ulnar physis and a second dog that had a hypertrophic nonunion of the femur, and the radius and femur of both dogs were harvested and cleaned of soft tissues. *[54 words in 1 sentence]*

> *Too short*: Two canine cadavers with orthopedic abnormalities were identified. The first dog had an unusual deformity. It was secondary to premature closure of the distal ulnar physis. The second dog had a hypertrophic nonunion of the femur. The radius and femur of both dogs were harvested. They were cleaned of soft tissues. *[51 words in 6 sentences; average, 8.5 words per sentence]*

> *A readable balance*: Two canine cadavers with orthopedic abnormalities were identified. The first dog had an unusual deformity secondary to premature closure of the distal ulnar physis; the second, a hypertrophic nonunion of the femur. The radius and femur of both dogs were harvested and cleaned of soft tissues. *[46 words in 3 sentences; average, 15.3 words per sentence]*

Remember that guidelines refer to averages. Variation in sentence length and complexity helps sustain reader interest. A publication full of overly long sentences is difficult to follow, and may lose a reader entirely. A sustained string of extremely short sentences can be choppy and annoying.

Children commonly string together a web of sentences connected by *and* or *but*, hardly stopping to draw a breath lest they lose their audience. Writers often unconsciously do the same, unnecessarily linking loosely related thoughts with conjunctions, semicolons, or commas – and lose their audience as a result. When faced with overly long sentences in your own writing, locate the connecting words and punctuation. Separate the thoughts into independent sentences.

> *An overly long sentence with weak connections*: Exposed poults developed enteric disease and exhibited 21% mortality during the first 3 weeks but controls had no enteric disease and exhibited no mortality; 20-week-old exposed turkeys weighed 0.6 kg less than

controls and had a higher incidence of angular limb deformities and also had a greater incidence of rotated tibias and showed bowed tibias, while controls had a significantly higher measurement for tibial shear strength. *[69 words in 1 sentence]*

Separated at weak connections, then edited for wordiness: Exposed poults developed enteric disease with 21% mortality during the first 3 weeks. Controls exhibited neither enteric disease nor mortality. When compared to controls at 20 weeks, exposed turkeys weighed 0.6 kg less, had more rotated and bowed tibias and angular limb deformities, and showed significantly less tibial shear strength. *[49 words in 3 sentences; average, 16.3 words per sentence]*

Limit average paragraph length

Paragraph length and complexity also influence readability. A paragraph length of about 150 words has been judged to be optimal for a scientific article. A paragraph that covers more than two-thirds of a page when typed double-spaced usually should be shortened. Select a few representative paragraphs, and use the word processing program to check their word count.

A paragraph that is too long and complicated is tedious to read. Reexamine the paragraph to see whether it includes more than one idea; often it will. Divide the paragraph between ideas. If paragraphs in a scientific publication consistently include fewer than 50 words (five average typewritten lines), they may seem scrappy and annoying to readers. Re-examine the text to see which paragraphs could be combined.

Present ideas in expected word order

In the English language, changing the word order clearly changes the meaning:

Hunter kills bear.
Bear kills hunter.

Proper word order is obviously needed to provide the intended meaning. In addition, studies have shown that people's ease in reading and understanding sentences depends to a surprising degree upon the grammatical order in which words appear.

The use of standard and expected word order – subject, verb, object, or SVO – makes ideas easy to follow because the words appear in the sequence in which things happen. When one writes "The cow swallowed a magnet," the reader mentally follows the action, seeing the cow, then the swallowing motion, and then the magnet, the object being swallowed. If instead, one writes "A magnet was swallowed by the cow," the reader unconsciously unscrambles the backward construction, converting it back into SVO order before grasping it fully. This takes extra mental energy and always interferes to some degree with effective communication.

Studying the works of 20 top writers (10 fiction and 10 nonfiction), Bjelland (1990) found that over 75% of their sentences used standard SVO order. However, in scientific writing, heavy reliance upon passive constructions results in an overwhelming number of inverted sentences. Change sentences back to SVO order whenever possible, while simultaneously keeping other aspects of readability under control.

Exercise 5–3. Readability

Improve the readability of these sample paragraphs by changing the sentence lengths and word order as needed.

1. The Haversian system consists of a canal in the center containing blood vessels and a nerve surrounded by concentric rings of bony matrix and between them scattered tiny spaces called lacunae filled with bone cells connected by canaliculi to one another and the central canal. Through this canal the cells are nourished and kept alive.

2. The kidney is a very important organ. It has the ability to secrete substances selectively. This makes it able to maintain proper composition of the blood and other body fluids. The various end products of metabolism are injurious if allowed to accumulate.

3. Sex-linked genes explain red–green color blindness in man, and if a woman heterozygous for color blindness marries a normal-visioned man, all of the daughters of this combination will have normal vision, but half of the sons will be color blind; however, half of the daughters will be heterozygous for the defect but the normal sons will show no trace of the anomaly and will never transmit it to their children; while the heterozygous daughters can have color blind sons, the homozygous daughters will never pass the trait on to their sons or daughters.

Uncouple long strings of nouns and adjectives

In English, a noun can be used to modify or describe another noun. Such noun clusters are common in our language, adding variety and flexibility to writing. For example, *heart disease* (a two–noun cluster) and *cardiac disease* (an adjective and a noun) have the same meaning, and may be used interchangeably.

Two-noun clusters are acceptable, even desirable, and usually cause no problems. However, scientists have a tendency to take this ability to extremes, running together whole series of nouns (and adjectives) that modify one another and the final noun in the chain, until the reader becomes lost. This construction – several modifiers stacked up in front of a noun – has been dubbed a "string of pearls." An excellent example which was actually published is this:

> Five two week old single comb white leghorn specific pathogen free chickens were inoculated with approximately 105 tissue culture infected doses of duck adenovirus. *[Which nouns are substantive and which are modifiers?]*

Strings of pearls often arise from an overly zealous attempt to be brief. However, lucidity is too important to sacrifice on the altar of brevity. Additional words and punctuation are preferable to barely comprehensible meanings. Suppose you encounter the phrase *aged dog meat samples*. It might have at least five meanings: samples of aged meat used for dogs, samples of aged meat from dogs, aged samples of meat from dogs, aged samples of meat used for dogs, and samples of meat from aged dogs. While this example may seem silly and extreme, similar examples are common in scientific writing. How would you interpret *brown egg laying flocks?* (It turned out that the eggs, not the flocks, were brown.)

Disconnecting strings of pearls is tedious but straightforward (Table 5.1). Working methodically through the typescript, circle every batch of more than two nouns. The goal should be to reduce these strings to simple pairs. As a memory trick, recall that "two is company, but three's a crowd." Because hyphenation links two words to reduce a three-word cluster to two, it often

Table 5.1. *Revising noun phrases that have long strings of modifiers*

Sentence fragment containing a string of pearls	How it might be revised for clarity
A system necessitated automated motor starting circuit	An automated motor-starting circuit required by the system
A 4 month secretory cell produced mucosal accumulation history	A 4-month history of accumulation of mucosa produced by secretory cells
The negative penicillin skin test result group	The group with negative results on the penicillin skin test
Blue absorbing pigment spectral curve	Spectral curve for blue-absorbing pigment
Climate controlled gene cluster phenotype variation	Climatically controlled variation in gene-cluster phenotype
Two dimensional real time ultrasonographic blood flow detection techniques	Ultrasonography techniques that detect blood flow in two-dimensional real time
A calibrated transit time ultrasonic blood flow probe cable end	The cable end from an ultrasonic blood-flow probe calibrated to measure transit time ultrasonically

bends this rule a bit. However, any cluster beyond two or three words usually spells trouble.

Decide the precise relationship of one word to another, and express this relationship by inserting necessary words. Start with prepositions, commas, and hyphens. Watch for unintentional changes in meaning. Noun and adjectival forms often have subtly different definitions (as in *paramedic training* versus *paramedical training*). Do not add an adjectival ending if the noun form more correctly expresses the thought.

Exercise 5–4. Strings of pearls

A.   Remove the ambiguity from the strings of nouns and adjectives listed below. Rewrite each at least twice to express different meanings clearly.

1.   mature muscle iron

2.   chronic depression symptoms

3.   renal lithium excretion

B.   Improve on the sentences below. In order to do so, you may need to assign a meaning to ambiguous phrases arbitrarily. More than one answer is possible; judge yours by its clarity.

1.   The three cases all had histologically confirmed metastatic malignant intra-abdominal tumors.

2.   The present study examines various immunospecific drug sample combinations and their inhibition producing effects upon human peripheral blood leukocytes.

Remove unnecessary hedging

To "hedge" is to protect one's arguments or statements with qualifications that allow for unknown contingencies or withdrawal from commitment. It also means to allow for escape or retreat. Whether from timidity, awe at the complexity of natural phenomena, or a misunderstanding of scientific "objectivity," scientists love to hedge (Table 5.2). In fact, double and triple hedges are common. However, each additional qualifier drains more force from the sentence. Sometimes the result is a sentence which says nothing at all.

> The cause of the degenerative changes is unknown but *possibly* one cause *may* be infection by a *presumed* parasite.

Table 5.2. *Some of the hedging words commonly used by biologists and medical researchers*

nouns	adverbs	verbs
supposition	presumably	appear
idea	probably	postulate
speculation	possibly	suggest
conjecture	apparently	seem
possibility	not unlikely	may be
inference	seemingly	speculate

One way of saying "I'm not sure" is usually enough in a sentence. When one hedging word is already in a sentence, prune away all the rest. However, if qualifying clauses must be used in a statement for accuracy, by all means include them. If there are many, consider itemizing them.

Exercise 5–5. Hedging

Reduce the following examples to a single hedge word apiece. Your interpretation of the sentence may influence which hedge word is kept.

1. These observations serve to suggest the probable existence of a possible female sex pheromone.

2. It seems that it might possibly be very wise to follow the outlined procedure.

3. Our belief is that the study may show an apparent link between cigarette smoking and lung cancer.

4. A possible cause-and-effect relationship is not unlikely.

5. The results appear to indicate that the mixture may have been more or less saturated with oil.

REVISE FOR BREVITY

Editor's creed

If you've got a thought that's happy –
Boil it down.
Make it short and crisp and snappy –
Boil it down.

When your brain its coin has minted,
Down the page your pen has sprinted,
If you want your effort printed,
Boil it down.

Take out every surplus letter –
Boil it down.
Fewer syllables the better –
Boil it down.

Make your meaning plain, express it,
So we'll know, not have to guess it,
Then, my friend, 'ere you address it,
Boil it down.

Skim it well, then skim the skimmings,
Boil it down.
Trim it well, then trim the trimmings,
Boil it down.

When you're sure 'twould be a sin to
Cut another sentence in two,
Send it in, and we'll begin to
Boil it down.

Author unknown

Editing for conciseness is both a matter of choosing the shorter, simpler alternative to express each word, phrase, and idea and a matter of eliminating redundancy. Wordiness is a common problem both within and outside the scientific community. Manuscripts are regularly returned to authors with the instructions, "Shorten this considerably before resubmitting it." Do not despair if this happens. A wide range of methods is available to edit for conciseness without having to remove significant material from the text. However, by attending to these matters before submitting the typescript, you may avoid that dreaded editorial directive entirely.

Beware of verbiage

Verbiage, which coincidentally rhymes with garbage, means the use of many unnecessary words. Often it leads to a sort of ritualistic, pompous writing style like this:

> Following termination of avian exposure, there was a substantial incrementation in lung volume and at this moment in time, it would appear that there has been a marginal degree of improvement in diffusing capacity. *[34 words]*

Even the most diehard among us would welcome with relief a shorter and more specific rewrite such as:

> After the man stopped keeping birds, his lung volume increased and diffusing capacity apparently improved slightly. *[16 words]*

There are no shortcuts around a fundamental step: Line by line and word by word, check through the first draft of the text. Ask "Is this word necessary? How can this be shortened? Does this say what I really mean?" Work on this point is not just an altruistic act directed toward readers. Practice directed toward simplifying expressions sharpens a writer's vocabulary and thinking skills.

Remove empty fillers

In spoken English, many words and phrases act as "fillers." They have little more meaning than *and-um* or clearing one's throat. Unless they are used to excess, neither the speaker nor his audience is even aware of them. In the lecture hall, a case for their utility can even be made – they pace a lecturer's talk to the slower pace of note-taking by listeners. In scientific writing, where each word should count, empty fillers have no place. Yet they sneak in, persistently and repeatedly. Certain of them are so common as to require special attention (Table 5.3). Most "it . . . that" phrases, such as "it is interesting to note that," are pointless fillers. Strike such phrases entirely. Particularly avoid those that contain thinly disguised double negatives. When equivalent alternatives exist, choose the one that takes the least space. This rule is, after all, the single idea behind all the more specific hints. A corollary, however, is that when clarity and brevity conflict, clarity is more important than brevity.

Table 5.3. *Examples of "it . . . that" phrases that can be removed or replaced*

Phrase with empty fillers	Shorter equivalent
It would thus appear that	Apparently
It is considered that	We think
It is this that	This
It is possible that the cause is	The cause may be
In light of the fact that	Because
It is often the case that	Often
It is interesting to note that	*omit*
It is not impossible that	*omit*
A not unlikely cause could be that	*omit*
It seems that there can be little doubt that	*omit*

Omit "hiccups" and other needless repetition

Short words (often prepositions) that unnecessarily accompany verbs or other parts of speech are sometimes termed "hiccups." Examples include "counted *up*," "faced *up to*," "check *on*," and "enter *into*." Omitting the italicized words does not change the meaning, a sure sign that the hiccup is unnecessary. A longer sort of hiccup occurs with roundabout, indirect constructions such as "There is a cure available. It consists of . . ." This can be rewritten simply as "The available cure consists of . . ."

Tautology, a closely related problem, is defined as needless repetition of an idea in a different word, phrase, or sentence. Poor scientific writing often includes many phrases in which one of the terms implies the other or in which one term in a phrase is in the general category to which the other term belongs (Table 5.4). For example, a *consensus* is defined as an agreement in opinion, so *consensus of opinion* is redundant.

Table 5.4. *Examples of tautology and hiccups; omit the italicized words*

Hiccups		Tautology
continue *on*	1 a.m. *in the morning*	*positive* benefits
refer *back*	at this point *in time*	*true* facts
check *up on*	collaborate *together*	large *in size*
all *of*	circulate *around*	many *in number*
true facts	*end* result	red *in color*
enter *into*	*mandatory* requirement	repeat *again*
face *up to*	*new* beginning	*past* history
	optional choice	*complete* stop
	five *in number*	prioritize *in order of importance*

A similar sort of wordiness occurs when words that are absolute are mistakenly modified. There is no difference between *absolutely complete* and *complete,* for example. Other absolute words that resist modifiers include *dead, extinct, fatal, final, honest, horizontal, impossible, inferior, libelous, lifeless, matchless, moral, mortal, obvious, peerless, perfect, permanent, rare, safe, straight, unique, universal* and *vertical.*

Some writers attempt to give their prose an air of elegance by using terms that contain two words which both mean the same thing. Common examples include *basic and fundamental; final and conclusive: null and void; each and every; first and foremost;* and *visible and observable.* Omit one word in each pair; the meaning is unchanged.

Shorten modifying phrases and clauses

Restrictive ("that") and nonrestrictive ("which") clauses have a valuable place in scientific writing (see page 148), but they are often overused. For shorter equivalents, replace "that" and "which" phrases with participles or other verb forms:

> *Wordy:* The organism that Chu (1993) found was a guppy that laid eggs.
> *Better:* The organism Chu (1993) found was an egg-laying guppy.

Scrutinize all prepositional constructions, especially those introduced by *of.* To reduce the length of wordy passages, substitute the adjective form of the nouns that are the object of these prepositional phrases. Alternatively, place nouns or noun substitutes in apposition.

> *Unnecessary prepositional phrases:* The dog with dysorexia was referred to a clinic in the neighborhood.
> *Better:* The dysorexic dog was referred to a neighborhood clinic.
>
> *Wordy prepositional phrase:* Group One includes a number of plants of the genus *Coleus.*
> *Nouns placed in apposition:* Group One includes *Coleus* plants.

Redundancy and verbosity are often coupled with jargon (see Chapter 7) and worn phrases which are so familiar that they pass unnoticed.

> *Verbose*: Due to the fact that breeder flocks in most cases are being subjected to periodical vaccination programs . . .
> *Better:* Because breeder flocks usually are vaccinated periodically . . .

When all these various kinds of changes are taken together, substantially shorter text can result:

> *Wordy:* The genera of the group of fungi that was studied by Fitzpatrick at this time are placed in the group of genera that are called the order Hypocreales because of the work of Miller (1941). *[35 words]*
> *Shorter:* The fungal genera studied by Fitzpatrick now are placed in the order Hypocreales because of Miller's (1941) work. *[17 words]*
>
> *Wordy*: The kitten which was the sole offspring of the calico was devoid of hair that was orange in color. *[19 words]*
> *Shorter:* The calico's sole offspring, the kitten lacked orange hair. *[9 words]*

Condense figure legends

Many journals prefer a clipped, sentence-fragment style of writing in figure captions; examine recent issues. Usually, articles (*a, and, the*) can be omitted and prepositional phrases can be treated as above, shortened, or omitted.

Full sentences: Fig. 1. The chromosome characteristics of the unknown strain of *Tetrahymena* are illustrated; notice the large and heavily stained object in the center of the photograph, which is the macronucleus. *[28 words]*

Clipped form: Fig. 1. Chromosome characteristics of unknown *Tetrahymena* strain; note large, heavily stained macronucleus (center). *[12 words]*

Exercise 5–6. Revising for brevity

A. How might one treat the following?

  1. It may be said that

  2. It has not been investigated but is possible that

  3. It is envisioned that

  4. It has been stated by critics that

  5. It is not irrelevant to mention here that

B. Identify and remove hiccups and other redundancy.

  1. It is interesting to note that the new organism is green in color, round in shape, 5 × 10 mm in size, and active with respect to motility.

  2. The authors envision that approximately 20–30 steps which are collectively referred to as electrophoresis will be necessary in the majority of cases.

  3. In the event that we hold a meeting at this point in time with reference to salaries, consensus should not be difficult to attain.

  4. The case load included 15 young juveniles and 10 mature adults.

  5. In this case, a viable alternative is quite unnecessary.

  6. Fig. 1. The lateral white cells as they have been shown to appear in a living abdominal ganglion of a cockroach. The ventral view has the anterior at top. The scale bar is 0.1 mm.

  7. The total absence of visible color was absolutely unique.

  8. To determine the mobility activity of the organism, new state-of-the-art equipment was used.

  9. For a full and complete understanding of the impacts and ramifications of the hot temperature upon the organism, it is our personal opinion that future plans should include a chilling procedure.

6

Checking grammar and number use

A dozen fumblegrammar rules for scientists

1. It is recommended by the authors that the passive voice be avoided.
2. Subjects and verbs even when separated by a word string has to agree.
3. Writing science carefully, dangling participles must not appear.
4. If you reread your writing, you will find that a great many very repetitious statements can be identified by rereading and identifying them.
5. Avoid using "quotation" marks "incorrectly" and where they serve no "useful" purpose.
6. The naked truth is that editors will read the riot act to any Tom, Dick, and Harry that uses clichés; avoid them like the plague.
7. In formal scientific writing, don't use contractions or exclamation points!!
8. If we've told you once, we've told you a thousand times, a writer who uses hyperbole will come to grief.
9. In science writing, and otherwise, avoid commas, that are, really, unnecessary.
10. Subjects and their verbs whenever you notice and can do so should be placed close.
11. Remember it is better not to, if you can avoid it, split an infinitive.
12. Proofread your manuscript carefully to be sure you didn't any words out.

Adapted from Safire (1990)

Proper grammar and number use are essential parts of effective communication, not only because they help avoid misunderstandings, but also because readers notice improper use. Fine points may be overlooked, but major errors distract readers' attention away from the primary purpose of the writing. No longer concentrating on the technical content, they start looking for more errors instead.

CHECK FOR GRAMMATICAL CORRECTNESS

The importance of grammatical correctness in scientific writing springs from the precision which science requires. Because more than one interpretation of a sentence or phrase is unacceptable, careful attention must be paid to both word choice and word arrangement. Most faults in grammar can be detected and corrected simply by analyzing sentences logically. Many books such as Hodges (1995), Strunk and White (2000), and Venolia (1995) deal more exhaustively with the details of grammar usage.

Decide whether active or passive voice is appropriate

"Voice" is the form of transitive verbs that shows whether the subject acts or is acted upon. When the subject of a sentence performs the action expressed by the verb, the voice is said to be active. When the subject undergoes the action of the verb, the voice is passive. The phrase *it was carried* is passive; *we carried it* is active.

The passive voice usually consists of some form of the verb *to be* plus the past particle of an action verb. (Forms of *to be* include *is/are, was/were, has/have been, had been, may be,* and *will be.* The past participle often but not invariably ends in *-ed* or *-en.*) Passive phrases include *were studied, is being considered,* and *will be examined.*

Who or what did the studying, considering, or examining? In the passive voice, the agent can be left unnamed. (It can, however, still be expressed with *by* if desired.)When the agent performing the action is unknown or irrelevant in the context, the passive voice is appropriate.

> Darwin's most influential work *was published* in 1859.
> Twenty-five genera of Capnodiaceae *are recognized* in the tropics.

The passive voice can also be used to emphasize something or someone other than the agent that performed the action. You might write *Johnson caught a fresh specimen* to emphasize Johnson or *a fresh specimen was caught by Johnson* to emphasize the specimen.

Use the active voice unless you have good reason to use the passive

Many scientists overuse the passive voice. They write as though it were somehow impolite or unscientific to name the agent of action in a sentence. They seem to feel that every sentence must be written in passive terms, and they undergo elaborate contortions to do so. However, in any type of writing, the active voice is more precise and less wordy than the passive voice. It is the natural voice in which most people speak and write. The active voice also adds energy to your writing, and forces you to decide *what* you want to say. The passive often obscures your true meaning and compounds your chances of producing pompous prose. Compare the alternatives in Table 6.1.

Table 6.1. *Active and passive voice*

Vague passive phrasing	Active, precise wording
It is recommended by the authors of the present study that . . .	We recommend . . .
The animal was observed to be situated in dorsal recumbence which had the effect of rendering its legs useless.	Lying on its back, the animal could not use its legs.
The data which were obtained by Johnson were probably indicative of . . .	Johnson's data probably indicate . . .
The following results were obtained . . .	We obtained these results . . .
It was discovered that a sustained coordinated effort will be required . . .	We need a sustained coordinated effort.

To convert a sentence that is in the passive voice to one in the active voice, search for the true subject, and name it. Then find the verb, and mentally drop the form of *to be*. Convert what is left of the verb to the active voice.

> *Passive*: The genetic relationship was studied by Berger and Shanks (1981).
> *Active*: Berger and Shanks (1981) studied the genetic relationship.

A more vigorous active verb also may be hidden in a noun ending in *-ion*. You can often exhume these buried verbs to convert the sentence into the active voice. For more help on this subject, see "Revise for Better Verb Choice" in Chapter 7.

> *Buried verb hidden in "-ion" noun:* Antibody detection was accomplished by Team A.
> *Resurrected verb:* Team A detected antibodies.

Check subject–verb agreement

Because of the writing style which they have adopted, scientists find it surprisingly difficult to use correct verb forms. The two most common grammatical errors in scientific writing are errors in verb use: subject–verb disagreement and dangling participles. Attention to subject–verb agreement is especially crucial because of the confusion which results from this sort of error:

> The effect of feeding rations containing concentrations of aflatoxin on the immune systems of young swine with lesions and enzymes were studied.

Were the effect and the enzymes studied? Or did the swine have both lesions and enzymes? Is *effect* the subject, in which case the *were* is incorrect? Because of lack of subject–verb agreement, the reader cannot be sure. The writers knew that the subjects and verbs must agree in number, but they allowed the two to become separated so widely that they lost track of them.

Exercise 6–1. Active and passive voice

Rewrite these passive sentences in the active voice. Condense and clarify the wording if you can.

1. It might be expected that this treatment would be effective.

2. No feed was available to the pathologist to analyze.

3. Inoculation was performed on 25 chickens by Jones and colleagues.

4. A collecting trip was made by this writer to Georgia for the purpose of collecting Lepidoptera.

5. Passages A and B should be marked for revision.

6. Two microscopes were reported stolen by the campus police last night.

7. Commercials have been prepared by the French government encouraging the use of condoms that are thought to be blunt enough to shock even liberal Americans.

8. A scientific writer's point must be clearly stated by him at the beginning.

9. If certain words are discovered to be missing from this medical dictionary, it must be remembered that no equivalents for modern technical words were to be had by ancient speakers of Greek and Latin.

10. Three incineration systems are being studied for the university president by administrative personnel at the Biology Building.

To check a sentence, temporarily omit all phrases that separate the subject and verb, including those that begin with such words as *together with*, *including*, *plus*, and *as well as*. This will give a sentence in which subject and verb are readily apparent. Both should be singular, or both should be plural. Correct the grammar, and move the subject and verb closer to one another to improve the sentence. For good measure, whenever possible also tighten the wording and recast the sentence in the active voice.

> *Incorrect grammar with separated subject and verb:* A high concentration of sialic acids which are a group of substances principally composed of amino sugars attached to polysaccharides, lipids, or proteins are found in the mammalian epididymis.

Omit intervening phrases: A high concentration . . . are found in the mammalian epididymis.

Improved, grammatically correct sentence: The mammalian epididymis contains a high concentration of sialic acids, principally composed of amino sugars attached to polysaccharides, lipids, or proteins.

Rewrite sentences with collective nouns and noun phrases

Most nouns are clearly either singular or plural in both sense and form. However, whether collective nouns are singular or plural depends on context and your emphasis as the writer. You must decide whether the action of the verb is on the group as a whole (and treat the noun as singular) or the action is on group members as individuals (and treat the noun as plural).

The pronoun *none* can also be singular or plural. When the noun that follows is singular, use a singular verb; when the noun is plural, use a plural verb. If you mean *not one*, use that phrase with a singular verb instead of *none*. Some examples appear in Table 6.2; consult a good dictionary if in doubt about the form of others.

Collective terms denoting quantity are particularly tricky to handle. When regarded as a unit, these nouns take singular verbs, but when considered individually they take plural verbs. We say "ten liters *is* a good yield" but "ten liters *were* poured into carboys." The problem is that, even with careful attention and the help of a good style book, such sentences often sound illogical or clumsy. Many writers simply prefer to redo such sentences. Write the sentence in the active voice and/or reorder it so the collective noun or quality is no longer the subject.

Instead of: Five milliliters of serum was added to the mixture.
Write: We added 5 ml of serum to the mixture.

Phrases like *a total of* can be particularly troublesome. *Total* is singular, and should take a singular verb. Do not say "a total of 35 animals *were* examined." Even the correct phrasing, "a total of 35 animals *was* examined," will cause many readers to stumble. It just sounds wrong! Usually the phrase *a total of* should simply be omitted.

Table 6.2. *Examples of verb use with collective nouns and the pronoun "none"*

Singular in context:	Plural in context:
A pair of animals was housed in each cage.	A pair of animals were watching.
All of the protocol was carefully followed.	All of the data were incorrect.
Statistics is a difficult subject.	The statistics are easily gathered.
The number of people in the study is dwindling.	A number of people have dropped out.
None of the information was used.	None of the trials were finished *OR* Not one of the trials was finished.

Remember that although the word *data* is sometimes used as a singular noun (particularly in nonscientific journalism), it is still correctly considered to be plural. (A *datum* is one of the single facts or pieces of information which collectively constitute the data.) Thus, in a scientific publication write, "Additional data *are* available."

Strings of subjects or verbs require special care

When the subject is composed of a singular and a plural noun joined by *or* or *nor*, the verb agrees with the noun that is closer.

> *Incorrect:* Neither the dogs nor the cat *were* in the cage when the assistant returned.
>
> *Correct:* Neither the dogs nor the cat *was* in the cage when the assistant returned. *OR* Neither the cat nor the dogs *were* in the cage when the assistant returned.

When a single subject is coupled with more than one verb, auxiliaries such as *was* and *were* can safely be omitted with verbs after the first. Many writers shorten sentences by doing so. However, a problem can easily arise when this condensing technique is used for a sentence with more than one subject.

> *Single subject, auxiliary verbs omitted:* Tissues were fixed in 10% buffered formalin, embedded in paraffin, cut, and stained with hematoxylin and eosin.
>
> *Two subjects, both plural, correct but confusing:* Samples were obtained from kidneys and sections cut and stained with lead citrate. *[Were samples taken from kidneys and sections?]*
>
> *Improved by removing one subject:* Kidney sections were cut, then stained with lead citrate.

If the number of the subject in the sentence changes, one must retain the verb in each clause. When two or more verbs are used with two subjects, one singular and one plural, keep the auxiliary words such as *was* and *were* with their verbs.

> *Incorrect:* The positions of the tubes were reversed and the test repeated.
>
> *Correct:* The positions of the tubes were reversed and the test was repeated.

Move misplaced modifiers

Whether they are single words or entire phrases, adjectives and adverbs must clearly refer to the word they modify. Because of poor placement in a sentence, misplaced modifiers appear to ambiguously or illogically modify an unintended word. To correct a misplaced modifier, move the adjective or adverb so that it is as close as possible to the word it modifies.

Exercise 6–2. Subject–verb agreement

Correct the following sentences if needed. Explain your reasoning.

1. The remaining fluid was drawn off and the kidneys washed.

2. Due to the small number of test animals used, that data was not significant.

3. Karyorrhexis, karyolysis, and cellular degeneration of hepatocytes was evident within the centrilobular regions.

4. The data indicates that Jones together with his wife and children was the first to discover the phenomenon.

5. None of the animals was harmed in the course of this study.

6. A sample was assessed by radiocarbon dating and sections analyzed by potassium–argon methods.

7. Neither the rats nor the chimpanzee were kept in the laboratory.

8. A total of twelve liters of serum were infused into the elephant.

Unclear: The researcher tested the women observing this schedule.
[Who observed the schedule, the researcher or the women?]
Better: Observing this schedule, the researcher tested the women.

Deal with dangling participles

Dangling modifiers have no reference point in the sentence. Participles are the undisputed champions when it comes to dangling. A participle is a verb form that acts like a hybrid between a verb and an adjective. It has some of a verb's usual features such as tense, voice, and capacity to take an object. At the same time, it also has features like an adjective, for it modifies a noun – denoting a quality, quantity, or extent of the thing named, or specifying the thing as distinct from something else in some way.

Most participles end in *-ing, -en,* or *-ed.* Examine the text for such clues.

Having euthanized the animals, we performed analyses.
Trapped by chlorophyll, light energy splits carbon dioxide, early scientists believed.

A participle is said to "dangle" when its implied subject is not the subject of the main clause of the sentence. Many dangling participles are misleading, confusing, or unintentionally ludicrous. To save face, locate them before readers do!

> Being in poor condition, we were unable to save the animals.
> Lying over the heart, you will discern a large growth.

The problem with dangling participles arises because the action is attributed to an agent that did not perform the action. The real sentence subject appears to be the subject of the participle as well. (Other parts of speech such as infinitives can also dangle, with the same result.) Consider this sentence: *Since first recognized in the 1960s many authors have described the syndrome.* The word *authors* appears to be the subject of *recognized*, although the writer intended the word *recognized* to refer to *syndrome*.

Two common "-ing" words are especially worth avoiding. One is *following*. Often it is used incorrectly to mean *after*. Following is a noun or adjective meaning that which comes next, as in "check the *following* reference" or "animals were examined the *following* day." It causes problems because it sounds like a participle to the reader. "*Following* a fat meal, the animal collapsed" sounds as though the animal was trailing the meal when this happened. Substitute the word *after*, which is clearly a preposition.

The other "-ing" word to distrust is *using*. It often dangles. Even when correct, *using* is a dull word which appears too commonly in scientific writing. Substitute a richer, more interesting word whenever you can. If you cannot think of one, at least substitute the safer word *with*.

> *Dangling participle:* No mosquitoes were found using the standard bait traps.
> *Better:* No mosquitoes were caught with standard bait traps.

Reliance upon the passive voice is a major reason why participles so often dangle. This is because the true subject is usually hidden in passive voice. Therefore, one straightforward way to correct a dangling participle is to rewrite the phrase to include the true subject of the verb which was turned into a participle. Alternatively, omit the verb of the participle entirely.

> *Dangling participle:* Using our inoculation procedures, infected hamsters developed granulomata.
> *True subject included, but wordy:* When we used our inoculation procedures, infected hamsters developed granulomata.
> *Verb of the participle omitted:* Our inoculation procedures produced granulomata in infected hamsters.

A third way to correct dangling participles is to switch to gerund phrases. A gerund looks superficially like a participle, because it also ends in *-ing*. However, a participle functions as an adjective, and a gerund functions as a noun.

Because a gerund functions as a noun, it often can be used as the subject of a sentence. When you say, "Writing is easy," the gerund is *writing*. (Sometimes gerunds also appear in the predicate part of a sentence, as in, "He explained the Kreb's cycle by *drawing* a diagram.")

Exercise 6–3. Dangling participles and other misplaced modifiers

Untangle the sentences below. Transform the sentences into the active voice when you can.

1. Progressing toward the anterior chamber a lamination was evident.

2. No bacteria were observed using dimethyl sulfoxide.

3. Following experimentation, bacteria multiplied.

4. Using this methodology the result demonstrated a correlation between the variables.

5. Intestinal sections can be examined for metazoan parasites using an inverted ocular.

6. Two stopwatches belonging to researchers that had been left leaning against cabinets were badly damaged.

7. For sale: laboratory table suitable for researcher with thick legs and large drawers.

Dangling participle: Flushing the flask, the impurities were removed.
Participle changed to gerund: Flushing the flask removed impurities.

Watch the grammar in comparisons

Most grammatical problems which occur with comparisons and lists arise from the omission of important words. When words are missing, the reader intuitively finds a parallelism among the words which are present. Strange, illogical comparisons sometimes result.

> *Nonparallel construction:* These results were in general agreement with others who found increased mortality. *[The results and "others" cannot logically agree with one another.]*
> *Parallel construction:* These data and others' results generally agreed.

The need for clarity always outranks the need for brevity. When comparing two agents under two conditions, fully specify which items are being compared. In the second part of a parallel construction, include all the words necessary to complete the comparison.

When comparing one person or thing with the rest of its class, use a word such as *other* with the comparative. Do not compare one with *all*, for it could be misinterpreted as the sum of the others.

Incomplete comparisons: Solution A yielded more amino acids than protein. The trial was significantly longer. The animal's weight was greater than all the others.

Completed comparisons: Solution A produced a greater yield of amino acids than of protein. The trial was significantly longer than the other trials were. The animal weighed more than any of the other animals did.

When comparing only two things, use the comparative term *(better, poorer, lesser, more)* rather than the superlative *(best, poorest, least, most)*.

Of the two medications, this is the *less* (not *least*) effective.
The brown dog was the *sicker* (not *sickest*) of the two.

Some words are not directly comparable because as "absolutes" they already represent the ultimate state – for example, *full, impossible, correct,* and *unique.* (See page 116.)

Incorrect: A more correct evaluation would say that our study was the most unique of its kind.

Correct A more nearly correct evaluation would say that our study was unique.

Watch your word order to be sure the word *as* or *than* is next to the comparing word. Look carefully when you have a phrase set off by commas or parentheses in the middle of the comparison. Check your grammar by omitting the phrase. Does it still make sense? Moving *than* and adding another *as* will correct the problem.

Incorrect: Group A was as large, if not larger, than Group B. *[Does "Group A was as large . . . than Group B" still make sense?]*
Correct: Group A was as large as, if not larger than, Group B.

Grammatical correctness and consistency are important for lists too

If there is an introductory preposition or article, either use it with only the first item or phrase in your list, or include it with every one. When some items take *a* and others take *an,* you must repeat the article with each item. (Remember also to put commas before conjunctions and between all items.)

Group 1 included a salamander, an alligator, and a skink.
Do not categorize clients by sex, by age, or by birthplace on these forms.
The patient's skin exhibited a red rash, an itchy lump, and a scar.

If a list is not inclusive, introduce the series of words or phrases with *such as.* Alternatives *like* and *e.g.* are less desirable. *Et cetera (etc.)* is rapidly falling out of favor, and at any rate, should never be used with these phrases.

Incorrect: Laboratory animals, like rats, mice, etc., were evaluated.
Correct: Laboratory animals such as rats and mice were evaluated.

Exercise 6–4. Comparisons and lists

Rewrite the following sentences to correct their comparisons and lists.

1. The authors' mild pulmonary hypertensive stage was similar to our present study.

2. In comparison to Group B, Group A was more unique.

3. The cat had a recovery that was better than the other cats.

4. The emergency medical kit contained a bandage, applicator, towel, brush, and a rubber sponge.

5. The fox was heavier than all the other animals in the study group.

6. Of the two alternatives, this is the most interesting.

USE TENSE TO SHOW THE STATUS OF THE WORK BEING DISCUSSED

The use of present or past forms of verbs has a very special meaning in scientific papers. Proper tense use derives from scientific ethics. The use of past or present verb forms is a way of indicating the status of the scientific work being reported.

Because of these conventions regarding tense use, a scientific paper usually should seesaw back and forth between the past and present tenses. An Abstract or Summary refers primarily to the author's own unpublished results, and uses the past tense. Most of the Introduction section emphasizes previously established knowledge, given in the present tense. Both the Materials and Methods and the Results sections describe what the author did and found. They appear in the past tense. Finally, the Discussion emphasizes the relationship of the author's work to previously established knowledge. This section is the most difficult to write smoothly because it includes both past and present tenses.

Use present tense when a fact has been published

Generalizations, references to stable conditions, and general "truths" should be given in the present tense. When scientific information has been validly published in a primary journal, it likewise becomes established knowledge. Therefore, use the present tense when writing about it. In this way, you show respect for the scientist's work. Similarly, when previously published work is mentioned, and the author is cited parenthetically or by footnote number, the sentence usually should be written in the present tense.

Serological tests commonly *are used* for the diagnosis of *T. cruzi* infections.

Several recent reports (2, 3, 6) *describe* similar findings.

The investigations of Graff (1932) *show* that the structure is a true perithecium.

This phenomenon *determines* the absorption coefficient of the tissue (Christensen et al., 1978).

When giving the author's name non-parenthetically as a source of the information, one can use either past or present tense for the verb that is linked to the author. However, the part of the sentence which refers to the scientific work itself is still given in the present tense.

Smith (1975) *showed* that streptomycin *inhibits* growth of the disease organism.

Jones (1978) *does* not *believe* that streptomycin *is* effective.

Use present perfect tense for repeated events

The present perfect tense is appropriate when observations have been repeated or continued from the past to the present.

Nesting behavior *has been studied* under many environmental conditions.

These drugs *have been shown* to produce significant elevations in blood pressure.

Use past tense to discuss results that cannot be generalized

Some results have been obtained under such specialized conditions that they pertain only to the particular study being reported. Numerical data sometimes fall into this category. Use the simple past tense of the verb that refers to the scientific work.

Barber (1980) reported that 28% of the 396 wasps in his study *showed* signs of parasitism.

It also would be correct to say "Barber (1980) *reports*," but using past tense for both verbs is somewhat smoother and more consistent.

Use past tense for unpublished results

By this line of reasoning, the research being reported for the first time in the paper you are writing will not be established knowledge until after it has been published. Therefore, use past tense to describe what you have done.

In the study presented here, the drug *killed* 95% of the *M. tuberculosis* bacilli.

Our data *showed* that few monarch caterpillars *survived*.

When your paper is published, the results become established knowledge. Thus, in citing your own previously published work, use the present tense, just as you do for others' work.

Use present tense to refer readers to your figures and tables

Even though these are new and unpublished material, they are explanatory aids, not research itself. Discussion of the research itself remains in past tense, but directives appear in present tense.

> Antibodies occurred in 11% of our mice, as Table 1 *indicates.*
> *See* Figure 3, which *illustrates* the six-fold increase in lutropin found in the study population.

TREAT NUMBERS CLEARLY AND SENSIBLY

Numbers are the heart and soul of most scientific research. If they are not reported clearly, a paper's value can be compromised or lost entirely. But while few dispute their importance, many are willing to debate fine points of how they best should be expressed. Should the number ten be written out or expressed as a numeral? Should large numbers be given scientific notation? What should be done with a series that includes numbers of very different magnitude?

One way to handle the situation is by edict. For example, many scientific journals now use Arabic numerals in preference to words for almost every situation in which a number is used. Check the *Instructions to Authors* for your intended journal, and follow their lead. Whatever style of expressing numbers you adopt, remember to be consistent.

Conservative rules determine when numbers should be spelled out

The most conservative style of scientific writing uses figures to express numbers 10 and above, and uses words to express numbers below 10 except when they are used as page numbers, as figure and table numbers, or with units of measurement. Several exceptions and instances of special usage expand on this rule (Table 6.3).

Numbers below 10 are generally written out, once again subject to a number of modifications (Table 6.4). Ordinal numbers, which express degree or sequence, may follow the same rules *(third, 15th)*. Alternatively they may be expressed as numerals whatever their size unless they are single words *(fourth, nineteenth, 44th)*.

When several numbers appear in the same sentence or paragraph, express them all in the same way, regardless of other rules and guidelines. Generally, Arabic numerals would be used whenever you have three or more numbers in a series, even if each of the numbers were below 10.

Exercise 6–5. Tense use

Indicate preferred tense use in the sentences below. If you feel that a sentence is correct as it stands, simply note the fact.

1. Recent work by Matthews (1980) showed that *Vespula* nests readily in the laboratory.

2. Bird size shows an increase in our study with width of wooded habitat, as Figure 2 indicates.

3. Beal (1960) also observed that size increased with meadow width.

4. In our study we find that there are significantly fewer antibody-producing cells in copper-deficient mice than in copper-supplemented mice (see Fig. 3).

5. In a study by Sengelaub and Finlay (1981), the average costal width for normal animals was 0.81 mm.

6. Conover and Kynard (1981) reported that sex determination in the Atlantic silverside fish was under the control of both genotype and temperature.

7. Recently published work by Fruchter *et al.* (1) characterizes the ash from the Mount St. Helens eruption of 18 May 1980.

8. Many researchers have confirmed that the balance of hydrostatic and osmotic pressures in the capillaries is a very delicate one.

9. ABSTRACT: The cell-to-cell channels in the insect salivary gland are probed with fluorescent molecules. From the molecular dimensions, a permeation-limiting channel diameter of 16–20 angstroms is obtained.

10. SUMMARY: Germinal and somatic functions in *Tetrahymena* are found to be performed separately by the micro- and macronuclei, respectively. Cells with haploid micronuclei are mated with diploids to yield monosomic progeny.

Table 6.3. *Conservative rules for situations in which numbers should be given as numerals*

General guideline	Examples
All numbers 10 and above.	Trial 14; 35 animals; 16 genera of legumes.
All numbers that immediately precede a unit of measurement.	A wing 10 cm long; 35 mg of drug; 21 days.
Numbers with decimals; fractions that include whole numbers.	7.38 mm; 4 1/2 hours.
Numbers that represent statistical or mathematical functions or results, percentages, ratios.	Multiply by 5; fewer than 6%; 3.75 times as many; the 2nd quartile.
Numbers that represent exact times or dates; ages; size of samples, subsamples or populations; specific numbers of subjects in an experiment; scores and points on a scale; exact sums of money; and numerals as numerals.	About 3 weeks ago, at 1:00 a.m. on January 25, 2000, the 25-year-old patients with IQ scores above 125 all awoke simultaneously in the nursing home at 125 Oak Street. They were paid $25 apiece to go back to sleep.
Numbers below 10 that are grouped for comparison with numbers 10 and above in the same paragraph.	4 of 16 analyses; the 1st and 15th of the 25 responses; lines 2 and 21.
Numbers that denote a specific place in a numbered series, parts of books and tables, and each number in a list of four or more numbers.	Trial 6; Grade 9 (but the *ninth* grade); the groups consisted of 5, 9, 1, and 4 animals, respectively.

> The 7 dogs, 8 cats, 9 mice, and 6 gerbils were exposed to applications of flea powder.
> The analysis revealed 22 complete answers, 4 incomplete responses, and 7 illegible ones.

Know when to combine words and numbers

Use a combination of figures and words to express rounded large numbers, starting with millions *(a grant budget of $1.5 million; almost 4 billion species)*.

Numerals and words are also combined when they appear as back-to-back modifiers *(two 13-ml aliquots)*. Generally it is best to keep the numeric form with units of measurement. Hyphenation minimizes potential confusion *(twenty 6-year-old patients* vs. *twenty-six year-old patients)*. If more than two numbers appear back-to-back in a string *(six 3–5 day intervals)*, rewrite the phrase *(six intervals of 3–5 days each)*.

You may spell out whichever number can more easily be expressed in words. Sometimes these combinations are awkward to read; in these cases, spelling out both numbers is preferred.

Table 6.4. *Conservative rules for situations in which numbers should be written as words*

General guideline	Examples
Numbers below 10 that do not represent precise measurements; numbers used in an indefinite, approximate, or general manner.	Five conditions; trials were repeated four times; a one-tailed *t* test; a three-way interaction; about thirty years old.
Numbers below 10 that are grouped for comparison with numbers below 10.	The second of four stimuli; five of eight living animals; in six cases, the disease lasted five times as long as in the other four.
Any number that begins a sentence, title, or heading (but reword to avoid this whenever possible).	Five patients improved, and 15 did not. Sixty-nine percent of the sample was contaminated.
Common fractions (those without whole numbers).	One quarter; reduced by half; a three-quarters majority.
The numbers zero and one when words would be easier to comprehend than figures, or the words do not appear in context with numbers 10 and above.	A one-line computer code; zero-based budgeting; one animal gave birth (*but* Only 1 in 18 gave birth).

> *Awkward:* The 1st three animals; the first 3 animals
> *Better:* the first three animals

Do not start sentences with numerals

When they begin a sentence, you must write out the number and unit in words, even if they would otherwise be written as figures. Revise such sentences whenever possible.

> *Incorrect:* 550 ml of hydrochloric acid should be added.
> *Correct but difficult to read:* Five hundred and fifty milliliters of hydrochloric acid should be added.
> *Revised:* Add 550 ml of hydrochloric acid.

Prefer Arabic numerals to Roman numerals

Roman numerals should be used only in certain stylized situations, such as the numbering of preliminary pages of a book or the tables in some journals, blood-clotting factors, or cranial nerves. At the same time, if Roman numerals are part of an established terminology do not change them to Arabic numerals. (For example, continue to speak of a *Type II error*.)

Arabic numerals are easier to read and interpret than Roman numerals are. Use them to number experimental research groups, organisms, virus types, and volume numbers in bibliographic material (even though Roman numerals may have been used in the original).

> group 3, echovirus 30
> case 3 in experiment 5
> blood-clotting factor VIII
> *Creative Acupuncture* 9: 6–35
> See the author's note in the preface (p. xiv).

For units such as weights, percentages, and degrees of temperature, use Arabic numerals. For example, write *3.2 m* or *72° F*, regardless of the way other numerical expressions may be treated. Unless a journal specifies otherwise, do not follow written numbers with a figure in parentheses representing the same number ("send three (3) copies to the editor"). However, it is both acceptable and desirable to include parenthetical material that amplifies understanding of other numerical data.

> He was given 2 mg of tetracycline on each of three occasions.
> A 10% mortality rate is common.
> Necrosis occurred in almost 20% (50/247) of the cases.

Use the SI metric system for measurements and weights

There actually are several metric systems, including the centimeter–gram–second system and the meter–kilogram–second system. However, these systems are gradually being replaced by a modernized metric system called SI, for *Système International d'Unités*. It provides unambiguous symbols that are standard in all languages (Young and Huth, 1998). The system is constructed upon seven base plus two supplementary units of measurement (Table 6.5).

Most scientific journals use the SI system and also permit some widely used units outside the SI system, such as liter, hour, bar, and angstrom. Most

Table 6.5. *SI fundamental units of measurement*

Quantity	Name	Symbol
Base units		
length	meter (metre)	m
mass	kilogram	kg
time	second	s
amount of substance	mole	mol
thermodynamic temperature	kelvin	K
electric current	ampere	A
luminous intensity	candela	cd
Supplementary units		
plane angle	radian	rad
solid angle	steradian	sr

scientific style manuals include a chart to convert measurements from traditional units to their SI equivalents.

All other units for physiochemical quantities are derived from these SI base units, though they may have special names and their own symbols. Prefixes join base units to express multiples. (Because kilogram, the base unit for mass already has a prefix, it is an exception. In this case attach the prefix to the unit stem "gram" rather than adding it to kilogram.)

For quantities much larger or smaller than a given base unit, standard prefixes are used (Table 6.6). The usual practice is to choose the prefix for multiples of 10^2 or 10^{-3} so the number accompanying the unit is less than 1000. Only one prefix may be used for most symbols, and a prefix is never used alone. Both the prefix and the unit it modifies are either abbreviated or spelled out.

> *Incorrect:* Add 6 μg of substrate
> *Correct:* Add 6 ng of substrate [or six nanograms]

When using SI, employ exponents for such expressions as *2 m²* (rather than *2 sq. m*). Avoid prefixes such as *hecto-*, *deca-*, *deci-*, and *centi-*, because they are not standard SI prefixes.

Table 6.6. *Standard SI prefixes*

Factor (power of ten)	SI Prefix	Symbol
18	exa	E
15	peta	P
12	tera	T
9	giga	G
6	mega	M
3	kilo	k
−3	milli	m
−6	micro	μ
−9	nano	n
−12	pico	p
−15	femto	f
−18	atto	a

Know how to express very large and very small numbers

Very large or very small numbers can be expressed in different ways. One is to use SI prefixes. Another is to use scientific notation. Check the *Instructions to Authors* and be consistent throughout the document.

> *SI prefixes:* 8,000,000 N/m² (force of newtons per square meter) becomes 8 MN/m² (not 8 N/mm² because the acceptable prefix should be attached to the numerator)
> *Scientific notation:* 8×10^6 N/m²

Often, a number can be rounded off without losing meaning. For example, 6,234,275 could be expressed as 6.2 million for most practical purposes. If a quantity must be converted to SI units, multiply the quantity by the exact conversion factor, then round it off appropriately. The format for reporting very large round numbers depends somewhat on the journal. In the absence of other specific instructions, substitute a word for part of the number (such as 1.5 million for 1,500,000). Because of usage differences between Europe and the United States, it is better to avoid the words *billion, trillion,* and *quadrillion.*

When reporting large but exact numbers, U.S. journals use commas between groups of three digits *(695,446)* in most figures of 1000 or more. (Exceptions include page numbers, binary digits, serial numbers, degrees of temperature, degrees of freedom, and numbers to the right of a decimal point.) For an international audience, do not break up numbers above 999 into groups of three digits with commas. In some countries, a comma indicates a decimal point. Instead, international journals often leave spaces *(695 446).*

The number of places to which a large decimal value is carried reflects the precision with which the quantity was measured. Omit nonsignificant decimal places in tabular data. One useful rule of thumb is to report summary statistics to two digits more than are in the raw data. For example, if scores on a test are whole numbers, report descriptive statistics to two decimal places.

Similar entries in a table row or column should be measured to the same level of accuracy, and the number of significant digits must be commensurate with the precision of your experimental method. The best level of precision for numerical data will vary, but rounded-off values often display patterns and exceptions more clearly than precise values.

Express percentages correctly

Three similar-sounding words confuse this subject. The term *percent* (sometimes written as two words, *per cent*) means "in, to, or for every hundred"; the symbol % can take its place. It should always be preceded by a number. *Percentage* means "a number or amount stated in a percent." *Percentile* is a statistical term for the value in a distribution of frequencies divided into 100 equal groups.

Except at the beginning of a sentence, use the symbol % and Arabic numbers for percentages. Repeat the symbol for each number in a series or range, including zeroes.

> These values were compared with the percentages for 1982.
> Ten percent of our students scored at the 99th percentile.
> The incidence of mononucleosis ranged from 0% to 24%.
> The bacteria were found in 15%, 28%, and 0% of the animals in
> groups 1, 2, and 3, respectively.

For purposes of comparison, percentages are often much more useful than an array of raw data. However, handling percentages properly can be tricky. One absolute requirement: whenever percentages (or other proportional figures) are employed, the finite number *(n)* from which the percentages are derived must be given somewhere. Often these numbers are presented in a separate column in the table.

Some authorities also recommend that the text include the actual number of subjects for each percentage if the cited series includes fewer than 100 subjects. They also recommend that you use decimals in percentages in series only when the percentages are based on more than 1000 subjects.

> Pulmonary disease was present in 50% (16) of the dogs, *OR* . . . in 16 (50%) of the dogs, *OR* . . . in 50% (16/32) of the dogs.

Whenever there might be a possibility of misunderstanding, state the basis for the percentages. For example, in reporting certain analyses, it may be essential to specify whether moisture-free ("dry") weight, fresh ("wet") weight, or volume was used.

Journals differ in what denominator magnitude (value of *n*) they will accept as adequate basis for a percentage. Percentages given for compared fractions with small denominators are likely to imply statistically significant differences when none in fact exist. In the example in Table 6.7, the percentages of drug-treated naive animals and drug-treated experienced animals look very different (60% vs. 80%), but in fact because of the small sample sizes, the real difference was only due to the differing behavior of a single animal.

Some clinical journals allow percentages only for fractions with denominators greater than 50. Thus, percentages would be given for the reader's convenience for 31/75 (41%) but not for 12/25. When some fractions would appear with percentages and others without them, it might be stylistically better to omit the percentages entirely. If differences in compared fractions are assessed statistically, the assessment must be based on the absolute numbers, not the percentages.

Report statistics sensibly and accurately

Statistical inference is an orderly means for drawing conclusions about a large number of events on the basis of observations collected on a sample of them. As such, it forms an important part of scientific inquiry.

All measures of variable biological parameters should be reported with statistical measures of this variability. In general, the sample mean and standard deviation or standard error of the mean (always appropriately labeled!) should be

Table 6.7. *An example of misleading use of percentages*

Group	*n*	Mating success (%)
Experienced	55	50
Naive, drug-treated	5	60
Experienced, drug-treated	5	80
Naive controls	25	41

stated. Medians and ranges may also be given, particularly if the reported data show a strong departure from normality.

As a biological or medical scientist writing for others in your field, be sure that both the text and table emphasize biology or medicine, not statistics. Statistical methods do not need elaborate presentation, nor do the mathematics of the test results need to be detailed. A simple statement of the chosen test and probability level is usually sufficient. Reference a basic text detailing the procedure if you feel readers might need it.

> *Poor:* To determine whether the two species differed in their egg cannibalism rate (Table 1), we used the Fisher Exact Probability Test, in which $P = (A + B)!(C + D)!(A + C)!(B + D)!/N!A!B!C!D!$, to obtain a $P = 0.56$ which was not significant.
>
> *Better:* The differences in the egg cannibalism rates of the two species (Table 1) were not statistically significant (Fisher Exact Probability Test, $P > 0.05$).

Whenever quantitative differences in data are reported that are found not to be due to chance alone, they should be accompanied by statistical statements that are the result of appropriate statistical tests described in the Methods section. In a table, these often are placed in a footnote. (Check format – some journals use letters for footnotes, others symbols, often with a prescribed sequence.) In the text, statistical results are usually presented in a concise style consistent with standard statistics books (ANOVA: $F_{111} = 7.98$, $P < 0.02$; Spearman rank correlation: $r_s = 0.81$, $N = 12$, $P < 0.01$).

Guard against statements that seem to imply value judgments about the results of statistical analyses with phrases like "nearly reached significance." Do not describe differences which are not statistically significant as *insignificant*! Likewise, avoid using the term *significant* to describe results when no statistical tests were run and you merely mean "important."

When statistical analysis was a tedious, largely hand-calculated affair, many a scientist shunned it entirely. Now, with the popularity of statistical analysis software, scientists face a strong temptation to overuse statistics, reporting strings of similar analyses or "massaging" data to an unreasonable degree. Almost nothing is more transparent than reliance upon prepackaged analyses without a corresponding understanding of their real meaning.

Use specialized symbols and notations sparingly and with care

In many scientific professions, communication depends heavily upon specialized notations such as symbols, equations, and formulas. These also are a type of illustration. They often appear on a line by themselves, like an in-text table. If complex, they may be submitted as a camera-ready photograph, like other artwork (see Chapter 4).

Scientific symbols and notations often express thoughts not easily or efficiently expressed as words. However, they have many drawbacks. They slow typing and word processing speed. They increase printing costs. And most

---

Exercise 6–6. Number usage and interpretation

Treat these sentences conservatively, spelling out numbers or changing them to Arabic numerals as appropriate.

1. A full 3/4 (75 percent) of the experimental animals died with 15 hours, but 17 horses (10%) were still alive forty-five days later.

2. The chemicals for the experiment weighed less than 1/5 of a milligram.

3. Approximately 20,500 cells were calculated to be affected.

4. The control group recovered more quickly but a chi-square test showed the difference was insignificant. We felt this was significant, however, because it showed the drug's effect.

5. The test plot contained ten species of grasses, two species of legumes, six species of trees, and 15 species of cruciferous plants.

---

importantly, they provide a stumbling block for audiences unfamiliar with them. Use such notation judiciously, explaining specialized symbols as necessary and carefully following the recommendations in a comprehensive style manual for your field.

Express mathematical formulations clearly. Short and simple equations, such as $x = 3y - 1$, should be set directly into the text, as done here. If a document has a great many equations which are referred to repeatedly in the text, they can be displayed (set on a separate line) and identified with consecutive numbers placed in parentheses at the right margin. For clarity, equations set off from the text need to be surrounded by space. Triple space between displayed equations and normal text. Double space between one equation and another, and between the lines of multiline equations. When a series of short equations appear in sequence, align them on their equal signs.

$$x(y) = (3y - 1)(z) \qquad (1)$$

$$p(x,y) = \sin(x + y) \qquad (2)$$

Entering over–under fractions can be a nightmare. Whenever possible, use a slant line or negative exponent to signify division, and change the format to a single line, like this: $(O - E)^2 / E^2$. If a really complex formula cannot be avoided, consider treating it like a figure. Furnish it in the form of a line drawing. In the same way, recognize that a symbol such as $\sqrt{\ }$ will cause printing problems that can easily be avoided by rewriting a phrase as "the square root of." Fractional exponents ($X^{0.5}$) may also be used instead of square root and cube root signs.

7

Revising for word choice

"When I use a word," said Humpty Dumpty, in rather a scornful tone,
"it means just what I choose it to mean – neither more nor less."

Lewis Carroll

How nice it would be if word choice were as simple in our own world. Instead, like the bugs that plague computer programs, flaws in word choice creep into scientific writing unnoticed (Weiss, 1990; Dupré, 1998). And as is true of the bugs in programs, there is more than one way to get rid of them. Like programmers, writers and editors may do anything to eliminate a bug – except add a new bug.

RECOGNIZE AND MINIMIZE JARGON

Jargon is a term derived from a medieval French word for the chattering and twittering of birds. It consists of highly specialized technical slang arising from the overuse and misuse of obscure, pretentious, or technical words or phrases. Often if spreads beyond the discipline in which it arose (as in the computer jargon in the preceding paragraph), and eventually, the changing English language may even fully embrace it. Until that time, however, a jargon word or phrase can pose an insidious trap for a scientific writer because its familiarity makes it seem acceptable before conservative usage embraces it as being correct.

Like other slang, jargon follows cycles of popularity, and fads are common. With a little reflection, you can probably add new examples to the ones we've listed in Table 7.1. Many of these arise by back formation, with a legitimate word or grammatical construction giving rise to illegitimate offspring. Modern dictionaries describe many of these words and phrases as "variants." This just means that many people are prone to the error.

When conventional words or phrases within a discipline are overused to create a verbal smokescreen, people call such jibberish "gobbledygook" and label it with the suffix -*ese*: legalese, educationese. A list of such terms could go on and on. Substitute shorter, everyday terms for polysyllabic synonyms of Greek, Latin, or Romance language derivation (Table 7.2).

Other gobbledygook symptoms that need treatment include a murky passive voice, endless strings of prepositional phrases, piled-up nouns, and parts of speech converted into other parts of speech. As Venolia (1987, p. 84) remarks,

141

Table 7.1. *Types of scientific jargon*

Origin	Examples
Careless extension of language rules	The kidneys were ground and the grindate was chilled.
	The material was rechromatographed.
	The mass was biopsied.
Acceptable words used in grammatically unacceptable ways	The substance was reacted with acetic acid. *(An intransitive verb such as "react" does not take an object, and has no passive voice.)*
	The feline developed leukopenia. *(Adjectives such as feline, canine, or bovine must have a noun to modify; when you mean cat, dog, or cow, say so.)*
	No histology was found in the liver. *(Histology's formal meaning is a discipline within the medical sciences; it is not a synonym for abnormality.)*
Spoken fads	Inoculize, prioritize, verbalize, visualize, or any such attempt to change a noun or adjective into a verb by adding "-ize." *(We have even encountered "formalinized samples" as a description of samples placed in formalin.)*
	Reactionwise, stepwise, or any such "-wise" except likewise.
	Phrases with "experience" tacked on the end, as in "a learning experience."
Words or phrases formed by dropping significant portions of a word or phrase	Prepped (prepared)
	Jugular ligation (jugular vein ligation)
	Osteopath (osteopathic physician)
	Vet (veterinarian)

"It appears there isn't a noun that can't be verbed!"

Eliminating jargon does not mean removing all technical terms, however. Technical terms are often polysyllabic, yet also concise because to convey their precise meaning in any other way would require many more words. When technical terms are used, be sure they are used correctly. Avoid using scholarly words or phrases in a pseudoscholarly way. Such jargon results in statements that are inaccurate as well as verbose. Words such as *spectrum, strategy, parameter,* and *approximated* have a meaning in the disciplines in which they arose. Used in a pseudoscholarly way in other disciplines, they can be misleading.

Watch out for spoken biomedical jargon

Biomedical terms can pose a special hazard because some are used incorrectly so often in speech that the misleading ring of familiarity can lend them false authenticity. Some examples follow.

biopsy – This is not a verb. (The mass was not "biopsied", but a biopsy of the

Table 7.2. *Suggestions to replace common overused words and phrases*

Instead of	Use
at this point in time	now
dorsal or lateral recumbency	on its back or side
due to the fact that	because
employ, utilize	use
high degree of accuracy	accurate
implement	do
in the event that	if
method	way
neonate	newborn
oftentimes	often
plethora	excess
postoperatively	after surgery
prior to	before
retard	slow
sacrifice, euthanatize	humanely kill or destroy
subsequent to	after
utilize	use

mass was performed). Observations are made on a biopsy specimen, not on the biopsy itself.

die of, die from – Persons and animals die *of*, not from specific diseases.

euthanatized, euthanized – Which of these words, if either one, should be used is a debated but unresolved matter; neither term even appears in some unabridged dictionaries. Use *humanely killed*, if possible. Avoid the term *sacrificed*, which has witch-doctor overtones.

parameter – Reserve this word for its specific statistical meaning of a potential variable to which a particular value can be assigned to determine the value of other variables. Do not use *parameter* to mean measurement, value, indicator, or number.

significant(ly) – Use only when statistical significance is meant, and give a *P* value. For other uses, change to *important*, *substantial*, *meaningful*, or *notable*.

Watch -ology *word endings*

The suffix *-ology* on words means the study of something. Words with this ending become jargon when used in sentences such as these.

> *Jargon:* No pathology was found.
> *Correct:* No pathologic condition was found.

> *Jargon:* Cytology was normal.
> *Correct:* Cytological findings were normal.

> *Jargon:* Serology was negative.
> *Correct:* Serologic findings were normal.

For example, "the only pathology found" translates into "the only study of pathogens found." It does not mean "the only pathogens found" or "the only tissue damage by a pathogen." Likewise, "etiology" is not a synonym of "cause" to be used in phrases like "the etiology of the disease"; it is the study and description of causes.

Note that words ending in *-ical* need an editorial check. Some editors drop the *al*, but others don't, as in *pathologic* vs. *pathological*. Be consistent.

Avoid coining new words, phrases, or usage

Rarely, a new scientific discovery truly justifies adding a new word to the language; if this happens, define the word carefully at its first mention in the document. Usually a little thought and dictionary work will produce an equivalent word that already exists in the English language. The work of translating a

---

Exercise 7–1. Jargon

A. Find a substitute for the following pretentious words and phrases.

   1. account for the fact that
   2. a sufficient number of
   3. has the capability of
   3. produced an inhibitory effect
   5. on a theoretical level
   6. on a regular basis

B. What do the following sentences literally mean? What did the author intend?

   1. The etiology of this disease is puzzling.
   2. Histopathology stages were based on ten dogs.
   3. The necrology confirmed the intestinal occlusions.

C. Reword these sentences to remove jargon and excess verbiage.

   1. The bovine was postoperatively traumatized by a defective electrified fencing enclosure, necessitating euthanatization.
   2. Positionize the slide carefully to visualize the quite unique spatial configurations with a high degree of accuracy.
   3. It is the author's opinion that it is not an unjustifiable assumption that this chemotherapeutic agent has the capability of significantly ameliorating and attenuating the symptomology of the disease process.

Table 7.3. *Common online acronyms*

Acronym	Meaning
ASCII	American Standard Code for Information Interchange, a widely accepted nonformatted text style
FTP	File transfer protocol, a system used to download files from a server to your computer or vice versa
GIF	Graphics interchange format, a compressed image format generally useful for line drawings or images with a fairly narrow range of color
HTML	Hypertext markup language, a standard Internet text format recognized by most Web sites and browsers
HTTP	Hypertext transfer protocol, a system used by the Web to move data such as files
ISP	Internet service provider, a company or organization that maintains the computer server and software to broadcast and access Web pages and other Internet services
JPEG	Joint photographic experts group (named for the group that developed it), an image compression method that works best for images with a wide range of color, such as photographs
PC	Personal computer, a somewhat ambiguous term used either inclusively to refer to all personal computers or exclusively for only those that do not run on a Macintosh operating system
PDF	Portable document format, a file type that preserves page layout and formatting across platforms. Read it with Acrobat Reader which is freely available on the Web.
URL	Uniform resource locator, the address or path name to a page or object on the Web
.zip	The most common file compression format for Windows PCs, often used for files to email or download to a hard drive; the most common Macintosh equivalents are .sit and .bin

scientific paper is difficult enough without putting these additional stumbling blocks in the path of the foreign reader.

New grammatical constructions that arise by back formation are particularly suspect. These include such "counterfeit coins" (Weiss, 1990) as *administrate* for *administer*, *preventative* for *preventive*, *remediate* for *remedy*, and *deselect* for *reject*. Sometimes they become slightly silly, as when the legitimate word *attend* gives rise to *attendee* rather than *attender*.

If you must use computer jargon, use it appropriately

Jargon, acronyms, and abbreviations are proliferating with the digital age. To use electronic databases, websites, and other online information sources effectively, it is useful to become familiar with at least the rudiments of this vocabulary (Table 7.3). We anticipate that with time many of these terms will become widely accepted. For now, be conservative. Excessive use of computer jargon can easily come across as pretentious.

Many new compound words pertaining to technology have not yet found their way into standard dictionaries. How should they be punctuated? The iconoclastic approach of computer manual writers seems to be "when in doubt, close it up," and they are the ones introducing new terminology and coining new meanings. Thus these new compound words commonly appear without hyphenation. Examples include desktop, download, email, keyword, online, toolbar, website, wildcard, and workstation.

USE THE RIGHT WORD

The difference between the right word and the almost-right word
is the difference between lightning and the lightning bug.

Mark Twain

The list of almost-right words is endless, and computer spell-checkers and grammar programs are little help with this problem. To rid your own writing of such mistakes, there is no easy alternative to learning what the right word is.

Some would like to believe that any widespread practice of writing or speech will inevitably become acceptable, and thus conclude that there is no cause for criticizing anything if it occurs regularly in the writing of educated people. If everyone confuses *affect* and *effect*, won't the dictionary eventually allow them as synonyms? And if so, can't we use them now? In a word, no. Good scientific writing is conservative. It must be less volatile than speech.

Remember, the function of writing is to permit communication across time and space. Most of us would have trouble speaking Shakespearean English today, but we can understand the King James version of the Bible, even though the English was written 400 years ago. Americans, Jamaicans, and Australians may have difficulty with each other's speech, but they have almost no problem with each other's writing.

Watch out for commonly misused and confused word pairs

Words are not always what they seem. Use a dictionary when you write so that people don't need to have one on hand when they read what you've written. Be especially careful about words that look similar but mean different things. The English language contains a great number of words that are commonly misused or mistaken for each other. Some commonly encountered "devil pairs" are given below. This list is only a beginning, and no substitute for a good dictionary.

accuracy/precision – *Accuracy* is the degree of correctness of a measurement or statement. *Precision* is the degree of refinement with which a measurement is made or stated, and implies qualities of definiteness and specificity.

acute/chronic – Reserve these terms for descriptions of symptoms, conditions, or diseases.

affect/effect – *Affect* is a verb that means to act upon. The noun *effect* means outcome. (As a verb, effect means to bring about, as in "it will effect a change," an awkward phrase worth replacing.)

aggravate/irritate – When an existing condition is made worse, it is *aggravated*. When tissue is caused to be inflamed or sore, it is *irritated*.

as/like – Rather than "like we just mentioned," say "as we just mentioned." *Like* can mean many things, but *as* is the conjunction for all but the most colloquial use.

case/patient – A *case* is a particular instance. It can be evaluated, followed, and reported. A *patient* is a person who is under medical care. (Avoid calling an animal a patient.) A sick person not receiving treatment is not a patient, so one cannot speak of untreated or normal patients.

compliment/complement – *Compliment* means praise, but *complement* means to mutually complete each other.

continual/continuous – *Continual* means happening over and over. *Continuous* means occurring without interruption.

dose/dosage – A *dose* is the quantity to be administered at one time, or the total quantity administered. *Dosage*, the regulated administration of doses, is usually expressed in terms of a quantity per unit of time. (Give a dosage of 0.25 mg every 4 hours until the dose has been ingested.)

examine/evaluate – Patients, animals, and microscope slides are *examined*; conditions and diseases are *evaluated*.

follow/observe – A case is followed; a patient is observed. To *follow up* on either approaches jargon, as does *follow-up study*. However, in medical writing the use of both terms is increasing.

gender/sex – *Gender* is cultural, and is the term to use when referring to men and women as social groups. *Sex* is biological; use it when the biological distinction is predominant.

imply/infer – To *imply* is to suggest, indicate, or express indirectly. To *infer* is to conclude.

infect/infest – Endoparasites such as intestinal worms *infect* to produce an infection; ectoparasites such as fleas *infest* and produce an infestation.

infectious/contagious – *Infectious* means harboring an agent that can cause infection, or having been caused by an infecting agent. *Contagious* is the adjective that means the agent in an infectious disease has a high probability of being transmitted. Under some conditions, an infectious disease is not contagious.

necessitate/require – *Necessitate* means to make necessary. *Require* means to have a need for. A patient requires treatment. The treatment may necessitate certain procedures.

negative/normal – Cultures, tests for microorganisms, tests for specific reactions, and reactions to tests may be *negative* or *positive*. Observations, results, or findings from examinations and tests are *normal* or *abnormal*.

over/more than – *Over* can be ambiguous. (The cases were followed up over 2 years.) Instead, say *more than*. (The cases were followed for more than 2 years.)

prevalence/incidence – *Prevalence* is the quality or state of being widespread or common. *Incidence* is the rate of occurrence.

principal/principle – A *principal* is a leader; used as an adjective, it means highest rank. A *principle* is a fundamental truth or law. Sam Jones was the principal investigator on a grant to study biological principles.

regime/regimen – A *regime* is a system of management of government. When a system of therapy is meant, *regimen* is the correct term.

symptoms/signs – A conservative rule states that *symptoms* apply to people, *signs* apply to animals.

toxicity/toxic – *Toxicity* is the quality, state, or degree of being poisonous. A patient does not have toxicity. *Toxic* means poisonous; a patient is not toxic.

use/utilize/employ – Generally, *use* is the intended term; *utilize* suggests the discovery of a new, profitable, or practical use for something. The word *employ* is best reserved for putting a person to work.

vaccinate/immunize – Although these words are sometimes used as synonyms, they carry different implications. To *vaccinate* means to expose a person or animal to an antigen purposively in hopes of eliciting protective antibody. To *immunize* implies that exposure successfully elicited protective antibody. Not all vaccinated organisms are immunized.

varying/various – *Varying* means changing, but *various* means of several kinds.

while/whereas – *While* indicates time and a temporal relationship. *Whereas*, often the word the writer intended, has such meanings as "when in fact," "that being so," and "in view of the fact that."

Beware of "which" and "that"

Your manuscript is both good and original; but the part that is good is not original, and the part that is original is not good.
Samuel Johnson

Because this pair of words causes so much confusion, it deserves extra attention. Sometimes the words can be used interchangeably. More often, they cannot. A phrase or clause introduced by *that* is restrictive; it cannot be omitted without changing the meaning of the sentence. Such essential material must not be set off with commas. A nonrestrictive clause adds information, but does not limit what it modifies. Because it can be omitted without changing the meaning, it is set off by commas.

Technically, the word *which* can be either restrictive or nonrestrictive. One could write "dogs which were treated recovered" or "dogs, which were treated, recovered," depending upon the sense of the sentence. However, many scientists overuse *which* as a connective, perhaps in a misguided attempt to make their writing more formal. As a result, correct comma use suffers. This simple rule of thumb is almost always correct: use *that* without commas with all restrictive clauses and *which* with commas with all nonrestrictive clauses.

Exercise 7–2. Devil pairs

Place each member of the devil pair in the proper place in the sentences below.

A. Like/As:

The results of our study were _____ those of McGowen (1967). A significant number of study animals staggered _____ drunks do.

B. While/Whereas:

Young dogs are very susceptible to distemper, _____ older dogs are often immune. Cattle often develop respiratory disease _____ being shipped to market.

C. Varying/Various:

Clients often have ponds which may be of _____ sizes. Each group received _____ combinations of antibiotics over the study period.

D. Effect/Affect:

Although we gave penicillin and terramycin, the drugs had little _____ . The _____ of the treatment was minimal. Trypsin-catalyzed digestion has the _____ of converting the substrate to short-chained peptides. In double-blind experiments, researcher bias does not _____ experimental results.

E. Principal/Principle:

He resigned as a matter of _____ . The _____ effect of centrifugation was to separate cell types. The _____ of independent segregation is fundamental to genetics.

F. Complement/Compliment:

To determine the appropriate value, one must find the _____ of the angle. The authors would like to _____ Jan Jones on her diligent effort. In the replication process, DNA and RNA _____ each other.

Restrictive that *clause:* Dogs that were treated with antibiotics recovered.

Nonrestrictive which *clause:* The researcher's decision, which did not come easily, was final.

When we read the words *which* or *that*, we interpret such words to refer to whatever went immediately before them in the sentence. If either word becomes separated from its true subject, confusion results. To cure the confusion, move the *which* or *that* next to the word to which it refers. Alternatively, rewrite the sentence to avoid using *which* or *that*. (This is an especially desirable route if the sentence is very long and/or complex.) Consider breaking the sentence into smaller ones.

Potentially confusing: Tumors were palpable in the animals that remained. *[Which remained, the animals or the tumors?]*

Ways to clarify the meaning: In the animals that remained, tumors were palpable. *OR* Tumors that remained were palpable in the patients.

Exercise 7–3. Which and that

Improve the following sentences in whatever ways seem sensible and correct, paying particular attention to "which" and "that."

1. It is relevant to mention here that novel paleontological findings have uncovered the strong probability that the genus *Cantius*, an early genus of primates of a primitive nature, had a large pedal digit that could grasp and which possibly may have figured in the evolutionary scenario of all of today's more modern primates.

2. It should be noted that the use of low molecular weight dextrans should be avoided in these patients which appear to pass through the damaged endothelium of pulmonary vessels.

3. Occasionally a parasite will be noted by the client on a fish which is more worrisome to the owner than to the fish.

4. According to this interpretation it is then concluded by the authors of this present study that ten thousand five hundred tons of lead, that are in addition to the ninety thousand tons which are presently being emitted, will be emitted into the atmospheric envelope during the course of the next calendar year.

5. Our efforts did not result in the location of the proposal which was missing.

USE BIAS-FREE, INCLUSIVE LANGUAGE

Words, like Nature, half reveal
And half conceal the Soul within.
Alfred, Lord Tennyson

In recent years, people have become much more aware of the ways in which language shapes our thinking. Many thoughtful discussions of the topic have appeared, and many guidelines have been developed; for examples, see Schwartz (1995), Schaie (1993), Maggio (1991), and the American Psychological Association (1994).

To avoid charges of prejudice and insensitivity, language and visual aids must be accurate, clear, and free from bias. Just as you have learned to check what you write for spelling and grammar, practice reading over your work for bias. Cultivate at least three kinds of awareness: (1) noting potential bias in the kinds of observations and characterization being made; (2) recognizing the impact of various value-laden terms; and (3) being sensitive to certain biases that are inherent in the structure of the English language.

It is a writer's job to maintain the audience's willingness to go on reading the document. Readers who are offended are likely to stop reading. Test your writing for implied or irrelevant evaluations on the basis of gender, sexual orientation, racial or ethnic group, disability, or age. Try substituting your own group for the one being discussed, or imagining you are a member of the group you are discussing. If you feel excluded or offended, the material needs revision. Another suggestion is to ask people from that group to read your material and give you candid feedback.

Use language inclusively, specifying only those differences that are relevant

Precision is a necessity in scientific writing. When you refer to a person or persons, choose words that are accurate, clear, and free from bias. For example, some writers use the generic masculine exclusively. This offends many readers, because it seems to be based on the presumption that all people are male unless proven female. Using *man* to refer to all human beings carries the same implication, and is simply less accurate than the phrase *men and women*.

Another part of writing without bias is recognizing that differences should be mentioned only when relevant. Marital status, sexual orientation, racial and ethnic identity, or the fact that a person has a disability should not be mentioned gratuitously.

Be sensitive to group labels

In scientific writing, participants in a study frequently seem to lose their individuality. They are either categorized as objects *(the elderly)* or equated with their conditions *(the demented)*. (Matters are not improved by changing this to *the demented group*!) Do not label people by their disabilities. Broad clinical terms such as *borderline* are loaded with innuendo unless properly explained. Calling one group *normal* may prompt the reader to make comparison of *abnormal*, stigmatizing individuals with differences (*the lesbian group* vs. *normal women*). Likewise, do not use emotionally loaded adjectives, such as "stroke *victims confined* to wheelchairs." Substitute neutral wording such as "individuals who had a stroke and use a wheelchair."

Labels such as *Group A* are not offensive, but they are not particularly descriptive either. The solution that is currently preferred places the people first, followed by a descriptive phrase (such as *people diagnosed with schizophrenia*).

Guard against the perception of bias or prejudice

A great many *-isms* have been defined by groups and committees working to reduce perceived bias in language. For helpful overviews and inroads to the literature, see publications by groups such as the American Psychological Association (1994) and the International Association of Business Communicators (1982).

Of the various types of prejudice, we are probably most sensitized to racism and sexism. Any verbal or visual reference that presents racial or ethnic groups as unequal or excludes one group in favor of another implies prejudice. Although racist language in scientific documents is rare, visual aids often do not show the same sensitivity. Sexism includes any verbal or visual reference that presents men and women as unequal or excludes one gender in favor of another; it can take many forms, some of them subtle (Zinsser, 1998).

Find alternatives to sexist language

Though it may be unconscious and unintentional, sexism is common in scientific writing. Consider these examples.

> Hard-driving veterinarians in private practice should take more time for their wives and children.
> Fuch's endothelial dystrophy in man occurs with a predilection for aged females.
> The client's behavior was typically male.

Some people are also quite sensitive to nonparallel usage that seems to suggest an inequality.

> The study included 10 men and 16 females.
> The researchers were surprised to find so many cautious men and timid women.

Avoiding sexist language isn't always easy, because the English language lacks a gender-neutral singular pronoun. A writer always has options; listed below are six of them (adapted from Schwartz, 1995; Carosso, 1986; Anonymous, 1975).

1. Use a gender-neutral term when speaking generically of your fellow creatures.

> *Instead of:* man; mankind; manpower; man on the street
> *Use:* the human race; humankind, people; work force, personnel; average person

2. Be sensitive to alternatives in titles and salutations. When a good gender-neutral term is available, use it in place of a clearly gender-oriented title.

> *Instead of:* spokesman; policeman; stewardess
> *Use:* speaker, representative; police officer; flight attendant

3. Use plural constructions when you can. Often, it is possible to recast a statement in the plural, thus circumventing the need to use the third person singular pronoun. Avoid breaking the rules of English grammar, however.

> *Sexist:* A doctor should advise his patients.
> *Grammatically incorrect:* Every doctor should advise their patients.
> *Better:* Doctors should advise their patients.

4. Replace the third person singular possessive with articles. Avoid s/he, he/she, and his/her. These constructions look awkward and interfere with reading. If none of the other guidelines has been helpful, use the slightly less awkward forms "he or she" and "his or hers."

> *Instead of:* Have the scientist send his manuscript to Dr Blow.
> *Better:* Have the scientist send the manuscript to Dr Blow.

> *Instead of:* Each technician must be sure that s/he signs his/her time card.
> *Better but awkward:* Each technician must be sure to sign his or her time card.
> *Better yet:* Each technician must be sure to sign a time card.

5. Address readers directly. If you can do so appropriately, substitute "you" for the third person singular pronoun. A direct instruction or command also works in many cases.

> *Instead of:* If the veterinary researcher cannot mail in his samples, he should ask his assistant if she can do it.
> *Better:* If you cannot mail in your samples, ask your assistant to do it.

> *Instead of:* A nurse must be sure that she uses disposable syringes.
> *Better:* Nurses must use disposable syringes.

6. Use the passive voice. (Notice that this option is at the bottom of our list!)

> *Instead of:* Each conference participant should have received his schedule.
> *Better (but only marginally):* Schedules should have been received by conference participants.

Exercise 7–4. Handling language sensitively

Improve the word choice in these examples.

1. A researcher must be sure that he double-checks all his references.

2. The sample consisted of 200 Orientals.

3. The depressives and the epileptics reacted differently to the drug.

4. The policeman apprehended a female for jaywalking.

5. The ten ladies in the study included one who was afflicted with cerebral palsy.

6. Breast cancer is one of the oldest diseases known to man.

7. We need 14 females willing to man the project.

Avoid awkward coinage

Some people feel strongly that a writer should avoid using words that are gender-specific when the roles that they denote are not gender-related. These purists have gone so far as to coin new words for any term that is gender-specific, as in substituting *parentboard* for the computer's *motherboard*. In the words of Dupré (1998), "even if the word is awkward, it shows your reader you are sensitive."

Or does it simply make you look silly? Experimental ways of making English more neutral have not caught on very well. Many commentators vehemently argue against artificial tampering with words. So-called political correctness, an attitude which carries language sensitivity to an extreme, has come under a great deal of public ridicule. Our advice is to take the middle ground. Use gender-neutral words when they are appropriate, be aware of nuances in our changing language, and avoid awkwardly coining new words.

REVISE FOR BETTER VERB CHOICE

Scientists are infamous for their plodding writing style. As a supplement to any other grammar-checking programs you may have – or as a fairly powerful checker on its own – consider using your computer's "search" or "find" command to flag the warning words and lazy verbs that appear in this section (or at least those you recognize as potential problems in your own writing). Each time that one is highlighted, examine the sentence in which it appears. You will soon become sufficiently sensitized that you no longer need the mechanical help to alert you to their presence so that you can avoid or fix them. As Weiss (1990) wryly notes, "Hardly anyone will say that your writing has improved. Rather, they"ll remark on how much smarter you seem lately."

Watch out for lazy verbs

Many scientists write as though only seven verbs exist: *demonstrate, exhibit, present, observe, occur, report,* and *show.* Certainly most scientific papers would be seriously crippled if these verbs were removed from the language. Consider this example:

> The mean hepatic weights *observed* to *occur* in normal and thyroidectomized rats were 154 and 27 mg, respectively. The kidney was also *observed* to *exhibit* a four-fold difference in the two groups, but as we have *shown*, no significant difference was *demonstrated* in the spleen. Figure 1 graphically *reports* these data.

All seven of these "lazy verbs" are overused, hackneyed, and trite. Whenever possible, substitute more vigorous verbs. Memorize the list to become alert to their appearance. Once you become sensitized to them, you'll be amazed to see how often they appear.

Furthermore, to be technically accurate, these lazy verbs should not be coupled with nonhuman subjects. For example, a scientist will write "the results demonstrate," which results, being inanimate, cannot do. Likewise, a researcher may say, "The tissue exhibited necrotic foci." A tissue cannot present anything for inspection, as the sentence literally implies. This misuse is so widespread that most readers have come to accept it. Nonetheless, this problem should provide additional incentive to substitute alternate wording whenever it can be done gracefully. The substitution will usually improve the writing in other ways as well.

> *Inaccurate:* Results show dog weight increased and reduced angulation occurred.
> *Better:* Dogs weighed more and angulation decreased.
> *Inaccurate:* As Figure 1 indicates, disease was seen to occur in 72 of the demented group.
> *Better:* Disease developed (Fig. 1) in 72 patients with dementia.

Unmask disguised verb forms

Habitual use of nouns and pronouns is a common cause of monotonous, verbose science writing. Abstract nouns formed from verbs and ending in "-ion" are a particularly common offender. Such words are really verbs in disguise, richer and more concise than the lazy verbs they are capable of replacing. They may be used directly as verbs or in their infinitive form. (For more help with this, see Chapter 6.) Experiment with adjectives, adverbs, and participles.

Overuse of abstract nouns: Following activity termination, the patient experienced an amelioration of his condition.

More forceful equivalent: After the patient stopped moving, his condition improved.

Buried verbal nouns: Results showed protection by the vaccine, but degeneration of lymphocytes occurred.

Resurrected verb: The vaccine protected the patients, but their lymphocytes degenerated.

Search for warning words

Sometimes, words which are perfectly good on their own still can indicate the potential for trouble. The words in this section are a case in point. The following "warning words" (adapted from Woodford, 1968) have remained relevant for decades; they usually indicate that unclear, ambiguous, or prosaic prose lurks nearby.

Colorless verbs – Like the seven lazy verbs, these are overused and lifeless. Colorless verbs occur most commonly as the past participle. They usually should be eliminated in favor of a more vital verb which is hidden (often in *-ion* form) in the sentence.

accomplished	achieved	attained	carried out
conducted	done	effected	experienced
facilitated	given	implemented	indicated
involved	made	obtained	required
performed	proceeded	produced	

Woolly words – These sometimes have a definite meaning. More often, they indicate that the thought needs to be sharpened. Think carefully about what is really meant, and shave the prose closer to its true message.

area	character	conditions	field
level	nature	problem	process
situation	structure	system	

Obscure antecedents – Pronouns are stand-ins for another word or group of words (their antecedents). What the pronoun is standing in for, or referring to, must always be clear to the reader. Ambiguous or obscure antecedents can be baffling or unintentionally humorous. Check the antecedent for such words as *all, it, its, this, that, their,* and other pronouns.

Vague qualifiers – Words such as *fairly, few, minimal, much, quite, rather, several, slight,* and *very* can and should be omitted, since they add nothing. Particularly watch their use with absolutes (such as "the animals were quite dead").

Dangling words – Remember that all words that end in *-ing* or *-ed* and all infinitives have the potential to dangle or be misplaced (see Chapter 6).

Exercise 7–5. Lazy verbs and warning words

A. Improve the following sentences in whatever ways seem correct and appropriate. Be alert for lazy verbs.

1. By early adulthood, more of the males than females were observed to exhibit severe symptoms characteristic of the occurrence of copper deficiency.

2. Under standard conditions, diazepam was chosen for inhibition of the initial rate of protein phosphorylation, as Figure 1 demonstrates.

3. The site of action of soap is observed to be at the cell surface.

4. Stanozolol caused prolongation of appetite, as the results demonstrate.

5. Isolation of *A. hydrophila* occurred.

B. Use infinitives to replace verbal nouns, and improve the wording of the following sentences.

1. The physicists' hope is for the solution of the question of whether science can harness alternative energy sources.

2. Transformation of the data was necessary for the statistical analyses relevant to resolution of the hypotheses.

SPECIAL TIPS WHEN WRITERS AND READERS HAVE DIFFERENT FIRST LANGUAGES

To think justly we must understand what others mean:
to know the value of our thoughts, we must try their effect on other minds.
William Hazlitt

Much scientific writing today has taken on a distinctly international nature. Communication between linguistic groups offers a special set of challenges. In this section, we offer some pointers for both the native English speaker writing for a reader with a different first language, and the writer whose first language is not English.

Translation is often touted as the answer. However, there is a shortage of qualified translators, and the expense can be prohibitive. Translation also delays the publication of scientific research. Furthermore, some languages have not developed the vocabulary required for science, so that in effect, translation requires the artificial development of terminology. Various software and online services promise translation, but as of this writing, not one has been refined to the point that they can be recommended for scientific documents.

Address second-language English readers effectively

At some point in your writing career, you may be called upon to write a document addressed to readers for whom English is a secondary language. Their task will be greatly eased if you pay careful attention to yours.

What MacNeil (1995) calls "the glorious messiness of English" has resulted in an estimated vocabulary of over one million words. (Other major languages have far fewer; French, for example, has only about 75,000.) This massive vocabulary poses formidable obstacles to those attempting to master what has become, to a very real extent, the first truly global language.

To facilitate communication, various experts have proposed special assemblages of restricted vocabularies and grammar rules. One of these is Simplified English, defined as a subset of Standard English intended for science or technical communication. Its most extensive use is for instruction and maintenance manuals (Gingras, 1987; Sanderlin, 1988), but it deserves wider consideration for the biological and medical sciences as well. Many of the recommendations for Simplified English are equivalent to those outlined in this book to improve scientific communications between native English speakers.

Simplified English is both a vocabulary and a technique. It starts with a basic lexicon of fewer than 300 nontechnical words, grouped by function (with definitions) in a thesaurus. To this, one adds one's own limited list of terms required by the specific document, and includes their definitions in a glossary with example sentences. Each of these words must have only one meaning in the specified domain of discourse. Use of jargon, vernacular phrases, and abbreviations is discouraged.

Because Simplified English is designed with science in mind, using its reduced vocabulary plus target terms works surprisingly well for most purposes. Often, clarity is improved by the change.

> *Instead of:* Unless one implements the modifications, there is a potential for damage.
> *Write:* Make the modifications, or damage can occur.

Additional guidelines are designed to keep sentence structure as simple as possible. These include writing only in the present, past, and simple future tense; using the active voice; and using the imperative (command) mood. Sentences are to be kept below 20 words in length, and no more than one sentence in ten on a page should exceed 16 words in length. The less skill and training in English the intended audience has, the shorter the sentences should be.

For further guidance, including the lexicon and numerous examples of basic usage, see *Science and Technical Writing* (Rubens, 1992).

Choose an effective approach when writing English as a second language

For multilingual writers whose first language is not English but who choose that language of publication, three writing methods are common:

1. Draft the paper in English from the start, doing the best you can. This is the most desirable way, because it usually results in the most readable text in the least time.
2. Write the first draft in your own language, then translate it into English yourself. This takes longer, and is more apt to lead to grammatical difficulties and stylistic awkwardness.
3. Write the paper entirely in your own language, then employ a professional translator who is familiar with the terminology of your branch of science. This can be expensive. Learn whether you can include the translation fee if you apply for a research grant.

Whichever method you choose, find a friend or colleague whose native language is English to read the nearly completed paper and make suggestions. Make whatever changes are necessary for your message to be clear. Referees and editors will probably not mind correcting minor mistakes, but they will reject a paper if they cannot even decipher the text's basic meaning.

Learning to write well takes effort and practice, and writing well in a second language takes even more. This section offers suggestions in five areas that seem to cause common and persistent problems for nonnative writers – count and noncount nouns; definite and indefinite articles; the verbals (gerunds, participles, and infinitives); verb forms in conditional sentences; and decisions about word order. For further study, the references in this section are a good place to start; see also Yang *et al.* (1996). Another helpful resource, English for Internet <http://www.study.com> offers live chats, placement tests, and free English classes (which fill up quickly).

Fox Trot

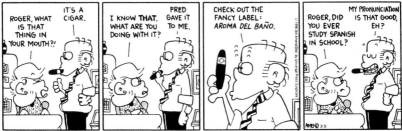

© Universal Press Syndicate.

Distinguish between count nouns and noncount nouns

Common nouns in English can be count nouns or noncount nouns. The distinction is important because it determines whether to use the singular or plural form of the word, and which articles *(a, an, the)* and limiting adjectives *(fewer* or *less, much* or *many,* and so on) to use (see below).

Count nouns refer to distinct individuals or things that can be directly counted. They usually have singular and plural forms: *gene, genes.* Noncount nouns occur as masses or collections of ideas that can be quantified only in a broad, vague way or with a preceding phrase. They usually have only a singular form: *mankind, honesty.* To confuse the situation, some nouns have more than one meaning; one meaning may be count, and the other noncount. *Water* is a count noun when we speak of a liter of water, but a noncount noun when we say that water is a limited resource.

When you learn a common noun in English, learn whether it is count, noncount, or both. Two dictionaries that include this information are the *Oxford Advanced Learner's Dictionary* (Hornby *et al.*, 1995) and the *Longman Dictionary of American English* (1997).

Watch use of definite and indefinite articles

The definite article *the* and the indefinite articles *a* and *an* are challenging to multilingual speakers. Many languages have nothing that directly compares to them.

Use *the* with nouns whose identity is known or is about to be made known to readers from general knowledge or some clue in the text.

> *The* amoeba's endoplasm spreads peripherally from *the* ends of *the* pseudopodium.

Use *a* or *an* only with singular count nouns. Use *a* before a consonant sound and *an* before a vowel sound. Pay attention to sounds rather than to spelling.

> *An* amoeba does not have cilia, but *a* protozoan often does.

This rule explains some of the differences between British and American English. The softer British pronunciation of an initial *h* in a word leads to *an historical,* but American pronunciation often accentuates the *h* and favors *a historical.*

To speak of an indefinite quantity rather than just one indefinite thing, use *some, less,* or *much* with a noncount noun. With a count noun, specify the number or use such words as *few, fewer, many,* or *several. More* is nice; it can be used with both noun types.

> *Many* unicellular animals can live without *some* sunlight.
> *Less* dietary vitamin C may mean *more,* not *fewer* colds.
> In *several* cases, the animals were unable to reuse *much* nitrogen.

Noncount and plural count nouns can be used without an article to make generalizations.

> Truth is beauty.
> Phenotypes may not reflect genotypes.

Many other languages such as Greek, Spanish, and German use the definite article to make generalizations. However, in English a sentence like *The fish are spawning* generally refers only to particular identifiable fish, not to all fish in general.

Watch gerunds, infinitives, and participles

There are three types of verbals: gerunds, infinitives, and participles. All three are derived from verbs, but function in several other ways. A brief review may help; see also Chapter 6.

A gerund is a verbal ending in *-ing* that is used as a noun. It can be used essentially the same way as any other noun. Only the possessive form of a noun or pronoun should precede a gerund.

> *Imprinting* is a widespread biological phenomenon. *[subject]*
> His *working* has not interfered with his *playing*. *[subject; object of a preposition]*
> Her primary research interest is chromosomal *mapping*. *[subject complement]*

An infinitive is the bare, uninflected form of a verb, without the restrictions imposed by person and number. It is coupled with the sign of the infinitive, the word *to*. An infinitive phrase consists of the word *to*, an infinitive, and any objects or modifiers. (It would be wise *to reevaluate our results*.) When an infinitive phrase begins a sentence, its implied subject should be the same as the subject of the sentence. Otherwise, it becomes a dangling modifier (see Chapter 6).

> *Dangling:* Not able to survive, the researcher discarded the bacteria.
> *Revised:* Because the bacteria were not able to survive, the researcher discarded the culture.

Knowing when to use infinitives or gerunds may be a challenge to multilingual writers. In general, infinitives represent intentions, desires, or expectations, whereas gerunds represent facts. (Other rules sometimes supersede this one, however.)

> *Starving* is the greatest threat for land animals. *[gerund describing biological condition]*
> They may travel long distances *to find food*. *[infinitive phrase describing intent]*

A few verbs can take either an infinitive or a gerund. With some (such as *begin* or *continue*) the choice makes little difference in meaning. With others, the difference in meaning is striking. A full list of verbs that can be followed by an infinitive and verbs that can be followed by a gerund can be found in the *Index to Modern English* (Crowell, 1964).

Understand participle use

A participle is a verb form that functions as an adjective. The present participle ends in *-ing* (exactly as a gerund does, the two being distinguished from one another only by their use). The past participle may end in *-ed, -t, -en, -n,* or *-d.* The perfect participle is formed with the present participle of the helping verb *have* plus the past participle of the main verb.

> *Present participle:* The *resulting* litter contained three kittens without tails.
>
> *Past participles:* The carcinogen's *known* and newly *discovered* properties should have alerted them.
>
> *Perfect participle: Having obtained* similar results before, the researcher stopped the trial.

Watch verb forms in conditional sentences

English pays a great deal of attention to whether or not something is likely to be a fact. Conditional sentences use the *if . . . then* construction with various combinations of verb forms to express the degree of confidence a speaker or writer has in the truth or likelihood of an assertion.

When a speaker assumes that what is stated in the *if* clause may very well be true, any tense that is appropriate in a simple sentence may be used. Use the same tense in both the *if* clause and the main clause. Adding the word *then* to the main clause is optional, but sometimes increases clarity.

> *If* this is true, *then* this must also be true.
>
> *If* you have conducted these tests properly, *then* you have already learned the answer.
>
> *If* pollen from a heterozygous plant is used, [*then*] you can show that the seeds have this genotype.

When predicting the future with some assurance, the main clause uses a form that indicates future time, but the *if* clause still must use the present tense (even though it, too refers to the future).

> This procedure *will be easier* if you *obtain* the proper glassware.

Suppose one has some doubt about the likelihood that what is stated will be put into effect. This is a time to use the past subjunctive, or *were to* + the base form, even though the *if* clause refers to a future time. The main clause has *would* + the base form of the main verb.

> If you *were to purchase* a new computer each year, you actually *would save* money.

A sentence that contemplates an impossibility uses the same "past tense for future time" rule, or a form that is even "more past": the past perfect in the *if* clause and *would* + the present perfect form of the main verb in the main clause.

If you *had lived* during the Jurassic Era, you *would have seen* dinosaurs.

Peruse prepositions and prepositional phrases

Words such as *to* and *from* are prepositions; they show the relations between other words. Not all languages use prepositions, and English differs from other languages in the way prepositions are used.

There is no easy solution to the challenge of using prepositions idiomatically in any language. Each of the most common prepositions has a wide range of different applications, and this range never coincides exactly from one language to another. For example, while Spanish uses one preposition (*en*) in all these sentences, English speakers say:

The bacterial cultures are *in* the incubator.
The petri dishes are *on* the laboratory bench.
Professor Jones arrives *in* the United States *on* January 15th.

English speakers often use prepositions as little more than space-fillers; see the section on "hiccups" in Chapter 8. These should be omitted.

She wrote *up* the laboratory report for all of us.
Better: She wrote the laboratory report for all of us.

Occasionally in English a preposition seems to have no object, but it is not a true hiccup because removing it changes the sense of the verb. Compare these sentences:

The fruit *drops off* the stem vs. The fruit *drops* the stem.

In such cases, the words that look like prepositions function instead as two-word verbs (phrasal verbs). Some of these phrasal verbs can be separated in a sentence, but others cannot. If in doubt, consult a comprehensive dictionary such as the *Longman Dictionary of American English* (1997).

Watch SVO word order

In Turkish, Korean, and Japanese the verb must come last, and languages such as Russian permit a great deal of freedom in word order. However, English sentences usually require a subject–verb–object word order.

Incomprehensible actual example: Depending on the course of study the student is taking, the SAT score and the GPA depending on the institution the student attends will vary.
Change to: Students' SAT scores and GPAs vary, depending on their institution and course of study.

Even when variations on this order are correct, they still make sentences more difficult to comprehend (see Chapter 5).

B.C.   by Johnny Hart

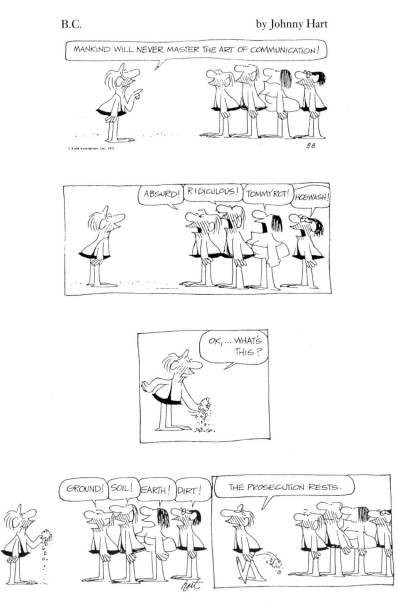

By permission of Johnny Hart and Creators Syndicate, Inc.

8

Revising punctuation and other mechanics

Confusion is always the most honest response.
Marty Indik

When journal editors or typesetters refer to style, they usually do not mean literary style. Instead they mean editorial style – the rules or guidelines a publisher observes to ensure consistency. Despite calls for standardization, nearly every journal details a slightly different set of requirements. However, none calls for other than correct usage on matters such as punctuation.

In this chapter we suggest ways of avoiding and correcting common mistakes that scientific writers of all nationalities tend to struggle with. If you feel the need for further advice on the finer points of punctuation and other mechanical aspects of editorial style, see general guidebooks such as Lunsford and Connors (1999), Shaw (1993), Strunk and White (2000), and Turabian (1996). Style manuals of special utility for biomedical writers include *Science and Technical Writing* (Rubens, 1992), *Publication Manual of the American Psychological Association* (1994), *American Medical Association Manual of Style* (Iverson, 1998), and *Scientific Style and Format* (Council of Biology Editors, 1994).

PUNCTUATE FOR CLARITY

Writing the words "a woman without her man is nothing" on the chalkboard,
the professor directed the students to punctuate it correctly.
The men wrote "A woman, without her man, is nothing."
The women wrote "A woman: without her, man is nothing."
Punctuation is everything.   *Author unknown*

Punctuation has one purpose – to help the reader understand the structural relationship within (and thus the intention of) a sentence. For this reason, the best approach to punctuation is almost always the simplest. Punctuation should be almost automatic. If you are puzzled over how to punctuate a particular sentence, you probably have created a sentence that will puzzle readers too, no matter how you punctuate it. Rewrite the sentence in a form that requires only simple punctuation.

165

Prefer the period

Semicolons, colons, and dashes indicate that two statements are closely related. Their use sometimes also helps condense material. However, sentences separated in this way are usually more difficult to read. The trend in scientific writing is to eliminate semicolons, and to use only periods to end sentences.

> *Older style*: A mutant strain might be designated "red"; its genetic symbol, *r*.
> *Newer style*: A mutant strain might be designated "red." Its genetic symbol would be *r*.

However, semicolons are appropriately used to separate items in a series with internal commas. (See page 167).

> Larval feeding habits of flies include: parasitizing beetles, moths, and other insects; mining in fern leaves, stems, and other plant tissue; burrowing in carrion, offal, and dung; and scavenging decaying vegetation.

Prevent false joining

Anytime a phrase would be nonsense without one or more commas, a dash, or parentheses, use them. This rule is the rationale behind all the more specific ones. When you have finished writing, check each sentence for reading errors associated with incorrect punctuation or lack of punctuation. If two parts might be joined erroneously, they should be separated by punctuation.

Pay particular attention to sentences which vary from the usual "subject–verb–object" word order. The possibility of erroneous joining is nearly always present when the introductory phrase contains a verb of some form, such as an infinitive or a participle.

> *Reading error possible:* Although additions of monensin were discontinued after 9 days the fermentors did not resume gas production.
> *Alternative interpretations clarified by punctuation*: Although additions of monensin were discontinued, after 9 days the fermentors did not resume gas production. *or* Although additions of monensin were discontinued after 9 days, the fermentors did not resume gas production.

Insert commas for clarity and emphasis

The comma has a wide variety of uses, but its overall role is to add clarity or emphasis to a sentence. Remember this fact, and the comma's many specific applications begin to fit into a pattern.

Whenever a dependent clause or a long adverbial phrase comes before the main statement of the sentence, it needs a comma. As an example, consider the previous sentence.

To determine whether to use commas with a clause that is within a sentence, read the sentence without the clause. Proper punctuation of a clause within a sentence hinges upon whether the clause is essential (restrictive) or not. If omitting the clause does not change the meaning of the main statement of the sentence, the clause should be set off by commas. If the clause is essential to the meaning, do not use commas. This rule generally means commas are used with the word "which," but not with "that." (See pages 148–150).

> The horses, which came from 6 farms, were dead.
> Six horses lived and 28 died. The horses that died were buried.

Punctuate the elements of series clearly

Series range from straightforward lists of like items to extremely convoluted sentences with all manner of nested phrases. For maximal clarity, they require different sorts of punctuation.

With a simple series, place a comma before the *and*, or the *or*, as well as between the items. Your composition teacher may have instructed you otherwise – in literary writing, and in United Kingdom scientific writing, this comma is often omitted on the grounds that it interrupts the flow of words. However, American scientific writing includes the comma, feeling it maximizes precision. Although the comma before the *and* is usually merely a nicety, sometimes it can be important to the meaning of the sentence.

Complex series need something more. When the individual elements in a series contain their own punctuation, separating the elements with commas may confuse readers. Use semicolons, numerals within the sentence, or both.

> *Confusing:* The criteria included that patients with unilateral dislocation were included but those with bilateral dislocation were not, as treatment of one hip may affect the untreated, and the child had to be less than 36 months old when treatment was begun and that no child with other anomalies such as scoliosis, arthrogryposis, or trisomy 21 was included.
>
> *Better:* All patients (1) exhibited unilateral, but not bilateral dislocation; (2) were younger than 36 months when treatment began; and (3) exhibited no other anomalies such as scoliosis, arthrogryposis, or trisomy 21.

Compound sentences can also be thought of as a type of series. Scientists are extraordinarily fond of coupling sentences, particularly when discussing their methodology. They also rely heavily on a single subject joined to pairs of verbs or adjectives. The words *and, but, for, or,* or *nor* are weak ways to join independent statements. Most critics of style shun them. Used to excess, such construction weakens the writing and creates a singsong cadence.

For stronger writing, examine each pair of sentences or compound predicates. First, consider dividing each statement into separate sentences, particularly if the statements are complex and/or long. Condense and tighten the wording. Then, if a weak connector still must be used, put a comma before it.

> *Weak writing, poorly punctuated:* Experimental subjects were kept in a climate-controlled room, and were provided with food. Artificial light was provided, and dogs were acclimated to handling. In the study described herein, the investigators found that *L. pneumophila* cannot multiply under these conditions but they do survive for they remain viable and this indicates that a great range of habitats is capable of harboring this bacterium.

> *Better:* Dogs were housed in a climate-controlled room with artificial lighting, provided with food, and handled. Under these conditions, *L. pneumophila* did not multiply, but they did survive, indicating that a range of habitats may harbor this bacterium.

Identify quoted passages from other texts

Any time you copy another writer's or speaker's exact words directly in the text, it must be set off in a way that shows it to be a quote. How this is done is determined by such factors as the quote's length (40 words or less is a common dividing point), the nature of the material being quoted, the country in which the document is being published, and both editorial and personal preferences.

Short quotes (called run-in quotations) are usually placed directly in the text, with quotation marks at their beginning and end. American and British styles for run-in quotations differ in their punctuation (Table 8.1). In general, U.S. and Canadian publications follow the American style, but U.K. and Australian publications follow the British style (Council of Biology Editors, 1994).

The American style is to use single quotation marks only for a quote within a quote. The names of articles or book chapters are treated the same way. If a run-in quotation is more than a single paragraph, begin each paragraph with a quotation mark but close only the end of the last paragraph with a quotation mark.

> Matthews states that "In his 1997 book, *Digital Literacy*, Paul Gilster quotes Vannevar Bush's seminal 1945 article, 'As We May Think,' and calls it 'the first visualization of hypertext in the modern sense.' "

> According to the CDC director, recurrent kidney disease is "unparalleled in this population."

> "If the hospitalization rate for this disease continues to climb as it has done this year, we are facing a problem of enormous proportions."

Longer direct quotes (called block quotations, excerpts, or extracts) may be set off as a separate block of type by indenting each line on the left side (in the same position as a new paragraph), and single spacing without quotation marks. The right margin stays the same as for the regular text. Sometimes the excerpt is set in a smaller font size than the main text. If the text that introduces the excerpt does not make its source clear, the excerpt should end with a parentheti-

Table 8.1. *Use of quotation marks in run-on quotations that appear within the text*

Context	American system	British system
To set off the primary quotation	Double quotation marks at the beginning and end	Single quotation marks at the beginning and end
To set off a quotation that appears within another quotation	Single quotation marks at the beginning and end	Double quotation marks at the beginning and end
Position of closing quotation mark in relationship to punctuation of the sentence	After a comma, period, exclamation mark, or question mark; before a semicolon or colon	"According to the sense" – before the punctuation except when the quotation is a complete sentence

cal indication of the source, placed after the closing punctuation mark of the excerpt.

> The problem of gobbledygook in scientific writing is serious. Gross and Sis (1980) offer this example:
>
> > It is envisioned that the bases for statistical analyses in this study will be predicated largely upon comparisons of the incidence (presence or absence) and/or the rates of incidence of histopathological conditions in samples acquired from primary platforms whose attributes have been carefully matched. (p. 127)
>
> These authors suggest a number of solutions.

With any direct quotation, be careful to enclose only the actual words used, not your restatement or interpretation. Follow the wording, spelling, and punctuation exactly. Whenever possible, verify the quotation from the original. To indicate an omission in quoted material, use three spaced periods (ellipses).

> Employees of the U.S. government may file a statement attesting that a typescript was prepared "as part of their official duties."
>
> Pauling stated that "Vitamin C . . . appears to be of . . . value"

Place other punctuation marks in proper relation to quotation marks. In American usage, the comma and period always appear inside quotation marks. The colon and semicolon are placed outside the quotation marks. Question marks and dashes go inside the closing quotation mark when they belong to the quotation, but outside when they do not.

> What did the author mean by "anti-rotaviral"?
> The term "pyrexia" is replacing the word "fever."
> Both the subjects and the researchers in the test were "blind," but the observers knew.
> We studied "mating readiness"; the other research team studied "recalcitrance."

Know when not to use quotation marks

Quotation marks are used in two different ways – to draw attention to words or phrases, or to attribute them to some other speaker. Do not overuse quotation marks for emphasis. Instead of using slang and colloquialisms within quotation marks, search for more exact terms and use more formal English.

In journals, quotation marks are often put around new technical terms, old terms used in an unusual way, or simply to draw attention to a word. (In books, italics are often used instead.) Used sparingly, these are acceptable when used to point out that the term is used in context for a unique or special purpose; in this way, they substitute for *so-called*.

Indirect quotations are paraphrases of a speaker's words or ideas. Do not enclose indirect quotations (usually introduced by *that*) in quotation marks.

> *Direct quotation:* Albert Einstein said, "Technological progress is like an axe in the hands of a pathological criminal."
> *Indirect quotation:* Jim Samuels said that he saw the sequel to the movie *Clones*, and it was the same movie!

Common nicknames, bits of humor, technical terms, and trite or well-known expressions (if they must appear) can stand on their own without quotation marks. Proverbial, biblical, and well-known literary expressions do not need quotation marks. Commonly known facts available in numerous sources need neither a source citation nor quotation marks unless the material is taken word-for-word from one particular source.

Hyphenation rules are complex and changing

Hyphens have two general purposes, dividing and compounding. They function primarily as spelling devices, but also can link or separate words or replace prepositions. Their most common use is to join compound words (such as *cost-benefit* analysis). They also form the compound numbers from *twenty-one* through *ninety-nine*, and fractions (such as *three-quarters*) when they are written out.

The decision whether to use hyphens with compound words – or omit them – often requires the aid of a good unabridged dictionary. The classical rules governing this set of uses are complex, covering such topics as whether the compound word is permanent or temporary and whether the words are so closely associated that they constitute a single concept.

As a spelling device, the hyphen is supposed to make life easier, but attempts to detail all its various uses tend to only increase the hyphenation confusion that many writers feel. In addition, the rules are changing, and even the authorities do not always agree. The use of hyphens in scientific writing clearly is declining. Although some rules still seem to generally apply (Table 8.2), there is a strong tendency either to form new single-word terms or to use strings of modifiers without hyphenation. Consult your intended publication for evidence of any

Table 8.2. *Ten hyphenation rules that generally apply*

Use a hyphen:	Examples
1. To create compound modifiers that precede a noun.	Pollen-bearing hairs; three-pronged structure.
2. To avoid ambiguity.	The food co-op bought a chicken coop; re-cover the cage so the birds can recover.
3. In compound numbers from 21 to 99.	Twenty-one, ninety-nine.
4. In fractions and ratios that function as adjectives.	A four-to-one vote; three-quarters gone.
5. To reduce redundancy in series.	The first-, second-, and third-born offspring were larger.
6. With letter or number modifiers.	5-week-old chick, H-bomb.
7. With strings of modifiers that express a single thought when the string comes before the noun, does not have an adverb as its first word, and would not make sense if each word modified the noun without the aid of the others.	Green-algae-covered ponds, scale-infested trees *but* freshly collected samples, a new digital analyzer, or equipment that is out of date.
8. With a prefix when the root word is a proper noun.	Pre-Darwinian.
9. When the same vowel ends the prefix and begins the root word (especially if *i* is the repeated vowel).	Anti-inflammatory; pre-existing.
10. Only when needed.	Unless misleading or awkward letter combinations result, the following prefixes may be used without hyphenation: pre, post, re, sub, super, micro, mini, multi, non.

strong prejudices, consult a standard dictionary for specific guidance, and then above all, be consistent.

Hyphens are also used to divide words at the ends of lines. Such divisions are made between syllables, but not all syllable breaks are acceptable end-of-line breaks. (Consult a dictionary.) Automatic hyphenation done by some word processing programs can produce some unusual word divisions. In general, it is best to turn off the automatic hyphenation option on such programs.

The main context in which this hyphenation role occurs is in the production of camera-ready copy. Much typesetting today is done in "ragged-right" style, with lines left unjustified so that the right-hand margin of the type column is irregular, but occasionally you may be asked to produce text that is "justified" (aligned to both margins). If justification is done with no hyphenation, the spacing between words is adjusted, sometimes to the extent of looking very strange.

When type is set in justified lines with hyphenation, it is inevitable that some words will be broken. Such text looks attractive, but it can be difficult to read. Furthermore, if a typescript is submitted in this style, there is a good chance that at least a few line-end hyphens may be carried over mistakenly as obligatory hyphens in the typeset copy. Unless your intended journal specifies otherwise, don't justify the text. By submitting ragged-right copy, you will minimize the chances of accidental erroneous hyphenation in the typeset copy.

Exercise 8–1. Punctuation

Correct the punctuation in these sentences.

1. Indicate optimum instrument settings for temperature humidity rainfall and performance.

2. When examined closely, the skeleton bears many bumpy spines, that project from the surface of the animal.

3. Class Echinoidea which includes sea urchins sand dollars and heart urchins is not closely related to class "Ascomyceteae."

4. The adults are radially symmetrical but the larvae are bilateral and it is generally held that this phylum evolved from bilateral ancestors and that radial symmetry arose as an adaptation to a sessile way of life.

5. The clinician asked, How did the patient die?; the answer was not obvious.

6. The essay, The Future of Veterinary Medicine, appeared in the early 1960's.

CAPITALIZE CONSISTENTLY

In general, all books and journals are using fewer capital letters than they once did. Still, to state all the rules for employing capitals would be nearly impossible here. (Capitalization rules in the 1984 *U.S. Government Printing Office Style Manual* cover 36 pages!)

Usage varies, and almost every rule has exceptions and variations. This confusion is more apparent than real, however. Most capitalized words are either proper nouns, major words in titles, or first words of sentences. However, a few problematic situations recur commonly enough in biomedical and biological writing to be worth special note in this chapter. If after reviewing the sections

Table 8.3. *Capitalization of proper and common nouns*

Proper noun	Common noun
Appalachian Mountains	the mountains
Eastern Hemisphere	the eastern world
Mesozoic Era	an ancient era
Celsius (scientist's name)	centigrade
Chemistry 605	chemistry class

that follow, you still have questions on capitalization of specific words, consult a standard dictionary and follow its lead.

Recall proper and common nouns

A noun that designates a specific person, place, or thing is called a proper noun. A noun that designates any and all of a class of persons, places, or things is a common noun. These two noun types differ in their capitalization requirements (Table 8.3). All proper nouns begin with capitals. Common names generally do not (except in special situations such as titles, see below).

Common nouns include chemicals, generic names of medicines, diseases, anatomical parts, or common names derived from the scientific names of plants and animals. When such names include modifiers derived from proper nouns, however, these modifiers are usually capitalized *(German measles, Darwinian finches)*. In the same way, capitalize the significant parts of the name of a manufactured product *(Pyrex glass)* and the vernacular names of plant varieties *(Yellow Dent corn)*. Capitalize the full names of government agencies, departments, divisions, organizations, and companies *(U.S. Department of Agriculture, Warner Communications Inc.)*.

Animal breeds are common nouns. However, in a paper mentioning several breeds of animals, capitalizing only modifiers derived from proper nouns gives the page a very uneven appearance Some writers and editors feel this lack of uniformity in capitalization is undesirable. They capitalize the full names of all breeds as a matter of equality. Be sure to examine a copy of your intended journal for examples of their policy.

> *Uneven capitalization:* The affected animals included Virginia deer, golden hamsters, and miniature Irish wolfhounds.
> *All breeds and species capitalized:* The second trial used French Poodles, Maine Coon Cats, and Parakeets.

Capitalize significant words in titles

Whether the title appears at the beginning of a work or is mentioned within running text, the role of capitalization is to help readers more readily distinguish a title from the adjacent text. There are various systems for doing this. Note that some reference systems for scientific and technical publications do not follow the usual guidelines, but have their own systems.

The classic system is to capitalize the initial letters of the first and last words of a title or subtitle, as well as all major (or "significant") words. Do not capitalize articles *(a, an, the)*, conjunctions *(and, but, if)* or short prepositions *(at, in, on, of)* unless they begin the title.

> For the test, be sure to read the book, *How to Write and Publish a Scientific Paper*, but for now you can ignore *The 1984 Summary of Wildlife Disease Reports*.

Some systems capitalize prepositions if they contain more than four letters *(between, because, until, after)*. Others maintain that only a word's function, not its length, should determine whether to capitalize it, and that even long prepositions such as *between* are most properly put in lower case, unless they are part of a phrasal verb.

> *Capitalization by preposition length:* She suggested that the participants should read the new book, *Weight Loss by Dieting Without Exercise*. See Turton's 1802 classic, *System of Nature After the Three Grand Kingdoms of Animals, Vegetables, and Minerals*.
>
> *Capitalization by word function:* His career really began with the publication of his insightful work, *Behavioral Interactions of Hospitalized Patients before and since the Arrival of Viagra*.

The first word of hyphenated compounds in titles is nearly always capitalized; the second word often is not, although either of these styles is correct. Some authorities capitalize the word following the hyphen only if it is a noun or a proper adjective, or if it is equal in importance to the first word. The word after such prefixes as *anti-, ex-, re-, and self-* may or may not be capitalized.

> *Aspirin and Anti-Heartworm Therapy*
> *The Role of Cancer-Inducing Agents*
> *Observations on a Hand-reared Baboon*
> *Short-term Goals and Long-term Management*
> *Self-measurements of Femoral Neck-shaft Angle*

All this seeming complexity and competition between systems may change with the popularity of word processing. Many programs include a case command with the option "title case" which capitalizes all words in the title automatically. Authors are all too ready to make the switch as soon as editors are ready to embrace it.

Check journal requirements

Some journals, publishers, and graduate schools specify a capitalization style; others don't. Make every effort to mimic the style of the journal in which you intend to publish. Examine recent issues. Note the figure legends, table captions, reference lists, and typescript headings and subheadings. You will probably find a definite capitalization style, even if one has not been spelled out formally in the publication's *Instructions to Authors.*

Capitalization is particularly variable in reference citations. Sometimes, article titles have the significant words capitalized. However, many journals prefer that article or chapter titles be treated as though they were sentences.

> *Capitalized article title:* Yalow, R. S. and S. A. Bernson. 1959. Assay of
> Plasma Insulin in Human Subjects by Immunological Methods.
> *Nature* 184: 1648–1649.
>
> *Sentence-style article title:* Guhl, A. M. 1968. Social inertia and social
> stability in chickens. *Animal Behaviour* 16: 219–232.

Exercise 8–2. Capitalization

Indicate accepted capitalization in the following sentences and titles.

1. The afghan hound ate plaster of paris.

2. The Study Sample included 15 greyhounds, 14 malamutes, and 10 spanish terriers.

3. adenine and guanine are nucleotides called purines.

4. A person can live normally without the Adrenal Medullae, but not without the Cortices.

5. these bacteria inhabit all Biomes of the northern hemisphere.

6. *A book title:* what's so funny about science? by sidney harris.

7. *The title of a scientific research paper capitalized by the "significant word" system:* assessment of the role of alcohol in the human stress response.

8. *A research paper title capitalized by the sentence system:* A Synopsis Of The Taxonomy Of North American And West Indian Birds.

KNOW HOW TO TREAT SCIENTIFIC NAMES

The scientific names of all animals, plants, and microorganisms are based on the rules set forth in the most recent edition of one of four codes, which authors and editors are obligated to accept:

International Code of Nomenclature of Bacteria. 1992. Washington, DC: American Society for Microbiology.

Virus Taxonomy: Classification and Nomenclature of Viruses. Sixth Report of the International Committee on Taxonomy of Viruses. 1995. New York: Springer-Verlag.

International Code of Zoological Nomenclature. 4th ed. 1999. London: International Trust for Zoological Nomenclature.

International Code of Botanical Nomenclature, adopted by the Fourteenth International Botanical Congress, Berlin, 1987. 1988. Konigstein: Koeltz Scientific Books.

Because of differences in usage and in the nature of the organisms themselves, the four major codes differ in some respects of terminology. For example, in botany a scientific name such as *Acer rubrum* is a "binomial" composed of a generic name and "specific epithet." In bacteriology, a name such as *Staphylococcus aureus* is a "binary combination." In zoology, *Homo sapiens* is a "binomen," and the specific epithet *sapiens* is a "specific name."

The codes also differ somewhat in practice. For example, the botanical code recognizes both subspecies and varieties. The zoological code also recognizes subspecies, but only those varieties named before 1961. The bacteriological code considers subspecies and varieties to be synonymous.

Additional useful references on bacterial nomenclature include *Approved Lists of Bacterial Names* (Skerman, 1989) and *Bergey's Manual of Determinative Bacteriology* (Holt *et al.*, 1994). Other helpful resources on biological nomenclature include Calisher and Fauquet (1992) and Jeffrey (1992).

Capitalize everything but species and variety

The basic systematic categories (*taxa*, singular *taxon*) in all of biology are, in descending order: kingdom, phylum or division, class, order, family, genus, and species. ("King Phillip came over from Germany soused" is an easy, if irreverent, mnemonic aid.)

The scientific names of all of these taxa and any sub- and supra-divisions are Latin or Latinized forms. All but the species name are considered to be proper nouns.

Do not capitalize the name of the species (except for the very rare journal which requires it). Technically, the species name is an adjective or similar modifier of the generic name, rather than a full name in its own right. For this reason, the species name is never used alone. The same is true of varietal names. For example, you might write of the common house cat as *Felis domestica*, family Felidae, but would never refer to it as simply *domestica*. However, after first mentioning the name in full, you can shorten it to *F. domestica* if the context makes the meaning clear.

Underline or italicize names of the genus, species, and below

Word-processing programs commonly include italics. However, underlining (which cues the typesetter to use italics) is often preferred in a typescript because it is easier to read.

Do not italicize the names of higher taxa. Like the genus and species, infraspecific taxa such as subspecies or varieties are italicized. Names of cultivated varieties (cultivars) are not italicized when they are not Latin or Latinized, but are set off with single quotes.

> *Canis familiaris*, family Canidae
> *Tris tricolor* var. *hirta*
> *Lilium superbum* 'Calico'

Make the first mention a comprehensive one

The genus and species (and variety, if relevant) should be given when a plant or animal is first mentioned in a paper. The most conservative usage adds the name of the scientist who first officially described and named the organism in print. This author citation need appear only once in the text, and usually does not appear in the title. Some publications take this concept to the extreme, and also include parts of the higher taxonomic classification of the organism.

> *Musca domestica* L. *[The L. is for Linnaeus, one of the scientists so widely recognized that a standard abbreviation for his name is allowed]*
> *Prunus australis* Beadle is a common ornamental plant.

Note that the word *species* retains the *s* in both singular and plural, and that the plural of *genus* is *genera*.

> *Ixodes scapularis* is a species of tick known to transmit Lyme disease; other species of *Ixodes* may too. This genus is only one of several genera known to be involved.

When an organism has been identified only to the generic level, the abbreviation "sp." is sometimes used as a shorthand for "some unidentified species of." The abbreviation "spp." signifies "several species of." Neither should be underlined or italicized.

> *Zanthoxylum* spp. were abundant, but *Drypetes* sp. was apparently rare.

After this first mention, the organism may be referred to by its common (vernacular) name if you wish. In most cases, do not capitalize this common name.

> *Solenopsis invicta* Buren . . . *S. invicta* . . . the red imported fire ant.
> The oak, *Quercus velutina* Lamarck, is found in North America. A relatively large tree, *Q. velutina* is prized for its wood. Its common name, yellow oak, alludes to the inner bark color.

Exercise 8–3. Scientific names

Indicate how the following scientific names should be handled.

1. the parasitic wasp, m. atrata.

2. the dandelion, taraxacum officionale, family compositae, class dicotyledonae.

3. the honeybee, apis mellifera var. ligustica.

4. the human malarial parasite, plasmodium falciparum Bignami.

5. the starfish (asterias) belongs to class asteroidea, phylum echinodermata, in the section deuterostomia.

Any family name can be transformed to a vernacular name by dropping the initial capitalization and the terminal *-ae*. Any generic name may be used as a vernacular name as well; this practice is common in bacteriology. Generic names are neither italicized nor capitalized when used in the vernacular sense.

> The family Chironomidae includes biting chironomids.
> *Salmonella typhosa* is a deadly salmonella.

KNOW WHEN AND HOW TO INCLUDE TRADE NAMES

A manufactured item such as a pharmaceutical product sometimes has as many as three different types of names. One is its systemic chemical name, which is often complex. Another is a shorter, nonproprietary "generic" name. A third is a trade name, also called a proprietary name. This is the name a manufacturer or vendor gives to its product; usually such names are registered as trademarks.

If one manufacturer's product behaves significantly differently from other similar products, readers may need to know which one you used in order to duplicate your experimental results. In such a case, the trade name should be given somewhere (often in parentheses or in a reference or footnote rather than directly in the text).

Otherwise, scientific writing generally avoids trade names. In particular, brand or trademark names should never be used in titles or summaries. One reason is that their use makes it appear as though one is advertising products. Another is that while generic and systemic names generally stay the same, trade names often differ greatly from one part of the world to another. Furthermore, official trade names can be awkward to use, because many consist of a long string of words, some of which may appear in all capital letters. (For example, the full name for those widely known sticky tapes is BAND AID® Brand Adhesive Bandages.)

Distinguish carefully between trade names and common names

Knowing whether a generally used name is proprietary is important. Considerable money has been spent, and many lawsuits have been entered into, to enforce the recognition of trade names! The problem is that when a trademarked product comes into general use, the public often loses touch with the word's commercial origins (Table 8.4). Proper names or their derivatives begin to function as common nouns, and for a period of time both styles exist side by side. Eventually, to the dismay of the company holding the trademark on the product, the product name or a variant of it may become an English word in its own right. (Aspirin, nylon, zipper, and fiberglass are examples of such lost battles.)

Don't slip into the pitfall of using trade names as though they were synonyms for generic products or processes. Usually, a quick perusal of the packaging will reveal a product's status. For more help, see the most recent edition of the *Trademark Checklist* (U.S. Trademark Association, 1994) or telephone the International Trademark Association (212/768-9887).

Substitute generic or chemical names whenever possible

The use of generic or chemical names for products is usually preferred in the text and obligatory in titles and summaries. Generic drug names can be verified in the most recent edition of:

> *USP Dictionary of USAN and International Drug Names.* Rockville, MD: US Pharmacopoeial Convention, Inc.

This useful annual guide is considered the standard source for U.S. adopted names (USAN). It includes formal chemical names of drugs, trade names, previously used generic names, and code numbers for investigational drugs, as well as an appendix that details the rules for coining new names. Many other countries have similar means for establishing nonproprietary names (see Council of Biology Editors, 1994).

Chemical compounds mentioned in clinical papers can be identified either by a formal chemical name or by a shorter "trivial" (from chemists' viewpoint) name. An authoritative source for verification of these names is:

> Budavari, S., ed. 1998. *The Merck Index: An Encyclopedia of Chemicals and Drugs.* 12th ed. Rahway, NJ: Merck and Co.

Cite trade names correctly

Sometimes there are reasons why it is critical to include a trade name in the text of a paper. When this is the case, use the common name first, then the proprietary name.

Table 8.4. *Trade names that companies are working to keep from coming into general use*

Trade name	Generic name
Vaseline®	petroleum jelly or petrolatum
SCOTCH™ Magic™ Tape	transparent tape
SPAM® luncheon meat	canned luncheon meat
XEROX® copier	photocopier
VELCRO® brand fasteners	hook and loop fasteners
BOTOX® Purified Neurotoxin Complex	botulinum toxin
SPACKLE®	surfacing compound

Like variety names (Yellow Radiance rose), and some market terms (Choice, Prime), trade names should always be capitalized. (With two-word names such as "Sorvall centrifuge" only the first or "significant" word is capitalized.) At least the first time the product is mentioned by full trade name, one should include a suffix superscript of the symbol ® for a mark that has been officially registered with the U.S. Patent and Trademark Office or ™ for marks that have not been registered but which the manufacturer wishes to identify as its own. (However, many journals omit the symbol.) The symbol need not be repeated in subsequent uses of the trade name. For example, write "the carrier ampholyte, Ampholine®" first, then just "Ampholine" or "ampholyte."

Include the manufacturer's name and address. Often this information is treated as a footnote. (Sometimes the trade name is included in a footnote and omitted entirely from the text.)

> Diets were supplemented with a multi-vitamin tablet (Preventron®).[1] Although other tablets were tried, Preventron tablets were most easily assimilated.
>
> [1]Natural Sales Co., Pittsburgh, PA.

WATCH FOREIGN WORDS AND PHRASES

Many words from other languages have been incorporated into the English language. In many cases, this happened so long ago that we no longer even recognize their foreign origin. These words seldom are an issue. The problem comes when words and phrases that are recognizably foreign are used primarily as affectation, to impress readers rather than to make an idea clearer than its English language equivalent would.

Consider degree of assimilation

Words and phrases that have been fully assimilated into the English language do not need any sort of special treatment, although for a while they may retain their original accent marks (especially if they are of French origin).

Exercise 8–4. Trade names

A. Indicate the correct way of citing these products in a typescript. Include correct punctuation and footnotes.

   1. the ammonium hydroxide cleaning solution produced by Armour-Dial, Inc., in Phoenix, Arizona and called "parsons sudsy detergent ammonia"

   2. diethyl carbamazine citrate tablets called "decacide," produced by Professional Veterinary Laboratories in Minneapolis, Minnesota

B. Rewrite the following sentences to remove the incorrectly used trade names.

   1. After adding water, place the fiberglass cap on the pyrex pitcher.

   2. Please send a xerox of the figure that shows the sparrow building its nest with kleenex and scotch tape.

   3. Patients should not don rollerblades for at least an hour after receiving botox.

   4. The abandoned dog survived on spam and vaseline.

Foreign words and expressions that have not been assimilated fully (Table 8.5) should be italicized if printed, or underlined if typewritten. This rule is often bent, however. Scientific writing is clearly moving away from the use of italicized words and phrases. Find an example in the journal if you can, or reword the sentence to use a plainly English equivalent for the word or phrase.

Watch plurals, because their form also depends upon degree of assimilation. Latin words that end in -*a* are made plural by adding -*e*. Those that end in -*um* are made plural by changing the -*um* to -*a*. This can be confusing. Many scientists fail to pronounce and spell these words correctly, speaking of "one media" or "a single larvae."

> These data are consistent because each datum is independent of the others.
> Wasp larvae in general are common, but the larva of *Eumenes* is not.
> A microfilaria is a worm-like creature; heartworm microfilariae sometimes invade a dog's heart.

As foreign words become assimilated, their plural forms give way to English plurals. However, because science tends to be fairly conservative, the acceptabil-

Table 8.5. *Examples of changing acceptance of foreign words and phrases*

Still considered "foreign" enough to take italicizing and/or original pluralization		
	Singular	Plural
sine qua non	formula	formulae has become formulas
coup de grace	memorandum	memoranda and memorandums are both acceptable
per se	a priori	none
coup d'état (coups d'état)	milieu	milieux is becoming milieus
Nonitalicized scientific words from Latin such as mitochondrion (mitochondria), bacillus (bacilli)	serum	sera is becoming serums
Nonitalicized words from Greek such as analysis (analyses)	appendix, index	appendices is becoming appendixes, indices is becoming indexes

The second column header reads: "Becoming "assimilated" enough to drop the italics and change its pluralization"

ity of the English plural forms often differs with the type of publication and its audience. Thus, one journal may pluralize *calyx* as *calyces*, while another uses *calyxes*.

In biomedical writing, certain commonly used Latin phrases cause additional trouble because they most properly follow the noun they modify. These include *in vivo* (in the living body), *in vitro* (in an artificial environment), *de novo* (anew), and *in vacuo* (in the absence of air or in reduced pressure). To place them before the noun, as though they were regular adjectives, is incorrect. Rather than "*in vivo* tests," say "tests *in vivo*." However, usage is shifting, and these eventually may be accepted as regular adjectives placed before nouns and without italics.

Prefer English equivalents over Latin and Greek abbreviations

An educated literary style once included the use of a number of Latin and Greek terms, particularly in footnotes. These are seldom seen in literary works today, and almost never in biological or medical publications. Avoid abbreviations such as *loc. cit.* (in the place cited), *op. cit.* (in the work cited), and *ibid.* (in the same work). For *viz.*, substitute "namely"; for *circa* use "about." The use of *etc.* (and so forth), while still acceptable, is rapidly falling out of favor; it commonly is not italicized.

The abbreviations below are still permissible, but are preferably confined to

---

Exercise 8–5. Foreign words and phrases

Indicate correct type use (italics or Roman) and format in the following sentences. Follow the most conservative route.

1. When acceptable, use the formulas already given in the book, *Official Methods in Microbiology.*

2. For information on the in vivo action of green plant pigments, i.e. chlorophyll, see Arnon's article in Scientific American and Calvin and Bassham's book, The Photosynthesis of Carbon Compounds.

3. Our experiments cannot identify the underlying biophysical alterations, viz., effects within the membrane itself.

4. Reduced oxygen tension provides the best environment for in vitro parasite development, as shown by Udeinya et al.

---

parenthetical references. However, their English equivalent is acceptable or even preferred. Punctuate as for their English equivalent. All these abbreviations are increasingly being used without italics and without periods.

> *i.e.* (*id est*, that is)
> *cf.* (*confer*, compare)
> *e.g.* (*exempli gratia*, for example)
> *et al.* (*et alii*, and others; note that the *al.* requires a period, but *et* does not)

MINIMIZE ABBREVIATIONS, ACRONYMS, AND OTHER SHORTENED FORMS

In general writing, use of shortened word forms may be decreasing, but in scientific and technical writing, abbreviations, initialisms, acronyms, and symbols are on the increase. You undoubtedly are already well steeped in their use in your own research field. Here we offer some brief guidelines and a plea for restraint. If they are not sufficient, entire chapters in common manuals are devoted to stylistic conventions for the many types of shortened word forms.

Avoid alphabet soup

Use abbreviations and acronyms sparingly and with discretion. They should be an aid to readers, not simply a convenience to the author. In particular, avoid using a string of either. This sort of shorthand is fine in a researcher's notebook, but not in a publication.

Use of IV 2-PAM and ATR lessened 1.5 LD_{50} OP toxicity at 3 h PO.

Some authorities decree that one should eliminate any abbreviation that is not used at least eight times in the text (including tables and figure legends). When a cumbersome name or phrase must be used frequently in the body of the typescript, first try replacing it with a pronoun or shortened version ("the drug," "the substrate"). Then go back and substitute abbreviations only where the text seems really to require it. Whatever abbreviations you use, make sure they remain uniform throughout your paper. Inconsistent abbreviations, more common than one would assume, are exceedingly annoying to readers.

Distinguish between abbreviations, acronyms, and initialisms

An abbreviation is the shortened version of a word *(temp., cm, avg.)*. Acronyms and initialisms are both formed from the initial letters or syllables of two or more consecutive words or each part of a compound term. An acronym is pronounced verbally as a single word *(NASA, ELISA)*. Each letter in an initialism is pronounced individually *(NSF, ATP)*. Theoretically, these distinctions should make it easier to apply rules of punctuation and capitalization to these forms, but sometimes they only add to the confusion because some authorities call initialisms a type of acronym, and others call acronyms a type of initialism.

The British distinguish further between true abbreviations (such as *diam.*, formed from the front part of a word, and requiring a period) and suspensions (such as *Mr* or *dept*, formed by removing the interior of the word, and in Great Britain used without periods). This British distinction has not caught on in the United States, but the general move to omit periods is becoming increasingly widespread. Periods are disappearing throughout the English language as it evolves. The best all-purpose rule is "be consistent."

> Doctor of Philosophy . . . Ph.D. or PhD
> United States . . . U.S. or US
> National Institutes of Health . . . N.I.H. or NIH
> amount . . . amt. or amt
> average . . . avg. or avg (preferred over ave.)

Shortened forms of capitalized words, and acronyms formed from them, generally should be capitalized and shortened forms of common nouns generally should not. Thus it is no surprise to find *SI* for *Système International* or *sp. gr.* for *specific gravity*. Exceptions include certain acronyms that have become accepted as common nouns *(laser, quasar, radar, scuba)*.

Initialisms take many forms. They may be written lower case (when generally they require periods) or upper case (when generally they do not require periods). Thus we have *c.o.d.* for *collect* (or *cash*) *on delivery*, but *TA* for *teaching assistant*. Many initialisms are written in all capitals without periods, even when the word itself is not capitalized. Thus we write *deoxyribonucleic acid*, but *DNA*. Internationally accepted biochemical abbreviations (*DNA, ADP, NADH*) do not need to be defined at first mention (see below).

To decide whether to use *a* or *an* before a shortened form, decide on a pronunciation rationale. Do not use an abbreviation or its plural form to denote a person by title or status. To do so is slang.

> *Incorrect*: Two MDs were consulted.
> *Correct*: Two physicians were consulted.

Use approved forms

Some technical, scientific, and industrial groups have adopted specific forms of abbreviations. Internal and terminal punctuation marks are often omitted. Carefully note such matters as punctuation, spacing, capitalization, and spelling. Many journals include a list of permitted abbreviations under *Instructions to Authors*. Commonly accepted lists appear in many places, including the *Handbook of Current Medical Abbreviations* (1998) and *Medical Terms and Abbreviations* (1998). See also Baron (1988), Campbell and Campbell (1995), DeSousa *et al.* (1995), Jablonski (1998), and Leigh (1998).

The form and acceptability of abbreviations for dimensions, distances, time, degree, measures, and weights are particularly apt to vary somewhat from one publisher to another. Abbreviate these terms only when they follow numerals. (Note that SI metric measures are nearly always preferred, and usually required.)

In the reference list, abbreviate the journal names by the system used by your intended publisher. Examine recent issues, and check the journal's *Instructions to Authors*. Most biological and medical journals follow the abbreviations in the BIOSIS List of Serials (*Biological Abstracts*) or MEDLINE (*Index Medicus*). These generally are available in the reference section of science libraries and online (see Table 2.2 on pages 28–29). The systems differ slightly from one another in both spelling and capitalization, but single-word titles *(Science)* are always spelled out in full.

Define shortened forms at first mention

The first time it appears, spell out any term you want to shorten, then give the abbreviation, acronym, or initialism in parentheses. Thereafter use the shortened form. If the abbreviation appears in the abstract (not generally recommended), define it again, since this may be published separately.

> The whooping crane (WC) differs from a lattice boom crane. Observers of the WC must watch that they don't become confused.
> For a partial list, consult the International Union of Pure and Applied Chemistry (IUPAC). The IUPAC list includes only those . . .

> Cultures were grown in trypticase soy broth (TSB). After TSB was added to the flask, the cultures . . .

Even if a word or phrase is defined at first mention, readers who consult only part of a chapter or journal article may have difficulty deciphering the abbreviation. Many conservative authors spell terms out at their first appearance in each major section of the typescript.

Pluralize correctly

When dealing with units of measure, use the same abbreviations for singular and plural forms (*50 mg, 25 IU, 100 ml*). For all-capital abbreviations, form the plural by adding *s* without punctuation (*EKGs, IQs*).

An apostrophe normally indicates the possessive case (*the animal's bones*). It may also be used correctly to indicate the plural of words or lower case letters when adding an *s* alone would be confusing ("mind your *p*'s and *q*'s"). Omit the apostrophe when pluralizing all-capital abbreviations or numerals, including years.

> *Incorrect*: In the early 1960's, RCB's . . .
> *Correct*: In the early 1960s, RCBs . . .

The words *page* and *species* have special plural forms when abbreviated that sometimes cause confusion in scientific writing. One page is "p." (not "pg.") and many are "pp." (not "pgs.").

> Consult Smith (1999, pp. 10–48).
> As the author states, "Infection is a serious matter" (Jones, 1998, p. 5).

Watch the names of geopolitical entities

When they stand alone, names of geopolitical entities should be spelled in full. The abbreviation U.S. (which sometimes appears without spaces or periods) is an adjective, as in U.S. Fish and Wildlife Service. As a noun, spell it out ("wildlife conservation in the United States").

In lists, tables, and when combined in an address, the names of U.S. states, territories, and possessions may be abbreviated in standard ways (Table 8.6). The preferred form still is the conventional system. However, it is rapidly giving way to the two-letter postal code system specified by the U.S. government for use with zip-code addresses and shown here in parentheses. Whichever system you use, be consistent. Do not switch from one system to the other.

When in doubt, spell it out

Here is a quick summary of some places not to abbreviate. Unless an abbreviation is internationally accepted *(DNA, RNA)*, avoid using it in the title or

Table 8.6. *Standard abbreviations for U.S. states, territories, and possessions*

Ala. (AL)	Idaho (ID)	Mont. (MT)	Puerto Rico (PR)
Alaska (AK)	Ill. (IL)	Nebr. (NE)	R. I. (RI)
Amer. Samoa (AS)	Ind. (IN)	Nev. (NV)	S. C. (SC)
Ariz. (AZ)	Iowa (IA)	N. H. (NH)	S. D./S. Dak. (SD)
Ark. (AR)	Kans. (KS)	N. J. (NJ)	Tenn. (TN)
Calif. (CA)	Ky. (KY)	N. Mex. (NM)	Tex. (TX)
Colo. (CO)	La. (LA)	N. Y. (NY)	Utah (UT)
Conn. (CT)	Maine (ME)	N. C. (NC)	Vt. (VT)
Del. (DE)	Md. (MD)	N. D./N. Dak. (ND)	Va. (VA)
D. C. (DC)	Mass. (MA)	Ohio (OH)	Wash. (WA)
Fla. (FL)	Mich. (MI)	Okla. (OK)	W. Va. (WV)
Ga. (GA)	Minn. (MN)	Ore./Oreg. (OR)	Wis./Wisc. (WI)
Guam (GU)	Miss. (MS)	Pa. (PA)	Wyo. (WY)
Hawaii (HI)	Mo. (MO)		

abstract. Titles and abstracts are often translated into foreign languages, where readers may find the abbreviations perplexing.

Do not begin a sentence with an abbreviation. Do not abbreviate generic names when they are used alone. (*Drosophila melanogaster* or *D. melanogaster* is acceptable, but never simply *D* or *D. m*.) Do not abbreviate units of measurement when they are used without numerals. (Never write "Several ml. were added.")

Exercise 8–6. Shortened forms

The following abbreviations are used incorrectly. Why?

1. *A title:* Assay for TCGF Activity in SPAFAS Chickens in the U.S.

2. *An abstract:* The present study provides first evidence for the presence of TCGF in supernatants of Con A stimulated chicken spleen cells incubated for several hrs.

3. *A text sentence:* Con A stimulated BALB/C spleen cells were used to prepare TCGF preparations by the MF I and MF II methods.

4. *A table title:* Distribution of ATPase in El treated membranes expressed as μ/mg of protein and total U.

5. *A footnote:* Pheasants were obtained from hatcheries in Ala., TN, and S. Carolina.

Finally, do not abbreviate when confusion might result from doing so. If two words have the same abbreviation, both should be spelled out.

PRACTICING MIXED CORRECTIONS: A SELF-TEST

When writing or editing a typescript, one is confronted with a potpourri of grammatical and rhetorical writing flaws rather than neatly categorized sets such as those presented in a writing book or style manual. The self-test that follows is given as an opportunity for practice of this slightly more realistic sort.

Find the errors, comment on them, and write a corrected version of the sentences. Your interpretation of certain sentences may differ from ours, but responses should aim in the same direction – toward increased precision and clarity.

1. The authors conclude that there is evidence that the limiting diameter lies between sixteen and twenty angstroms in these cells taken from mammals.

2. The inhibitory activity of the various combinations was studied and isobolograms plotted.

3. The site of action of EDTA is at the cell surface by increasing cell wall permeability.

4. Measurements were made of the pronounced lesions that were in the heart.

5. Numerous strains of T. cruzi are reported to cause chronic *chagas disease*.

6. In the present study, treatment is terminated when fish appear irritated.

7. The wasp S. maculata is a progressive provisioner and transports the flies held ventrally by the middle legs.

8. Figure 24 is a cichlid fish from a Florida pond where metacercariae (at arrow) were found in the gill cavity.

9. You should mix 1500 ml of dye with 7,000 ml of water.

10. Fruits in the diet of Artibeus included an orange, pear, apple and peach.

11. Ichthyophthirius is one of the few parasites of fish with cilia.

12. The authors encountered amorphous material of varying density.

13. The animals were equally divided into 5 groups of 22 each.

14. Cotton swabs were obtained from tracheas.

15. Many of their published results indicated that perhaps MG organisms may be poorly transmitted at times.

16. The results were obtained from HPLC a useful technique for the analysis of aflatoxins in feeds with excellent resolution.

17. There is a possible cause which must be faced up to. It is in regard to whether aflatoxin enters into the blood stream.

18. An excessive amount of solar radiation received at a rapid rate has been shown by a large body of data to have the capability of inflicting epidermal damage.

19. When the horse was circled to the left and right, lameness was evidenced which was not cyclic but continual.

20. None of these dogs, that were housed in runs and were not challenged by exercise, developed any clinical signs of heartworm disease.

Selected references

Alley, M. (1987). *The Craft of Scientific Writing*. Englewood Cliffs, NJ: Prentice-Hall.
Alley, M. (1996). *The Craft of Scientific Writing*. 3rd edn. New York: Springer-Verlag.
American Psychological Association. (1994). *Publication Manual*. 4th edn. Washington, DC: American Psychological Association.
Anonymous. (1975). Guidelines for nonsexist use of language. *American Psychologist*, **30**, 682–6.
(1994). *The Author's Guide to Biomedical Journals: Complete Manuscript Submission Instructions for 185 Leading Biomedical Periodicals*. New York: Mary Ann Liebert, Inc.
Aslett, D. (1996). *How to Have a 48-hour Day*. Cincinnatti, OH: F & W Publications, Inc.
Atlas, M. C. (1995). *Author's Handbook of Styles for Life Science Journals*. 2nd edn. Boca Raton, FL: CRC Press.
Baron, D. N. (1988). *Units, Symbols, and Abbreviations: A Guide for Biological and Medical Editors*. 4th edn. London: Royal Society of Medicine.
Benson, B. W. & Boege, S. (1999). *Handbook of Good Laboratory Practices*. Bristol, PA: Hemisphere Publishing.
Bjelland, H. (1990). *Writing Better Technical Articles*. Blue Ridge Summit, PA: TAB Books.
Blanchard, D. C. (1974). References and unreferences. *Science*, **185**, 1003.
Blum, D. & Knudson, M. (eds.). (1997). *A Field Guide for Science Writers*. New York: Oxford University Press.
Bolker, J. (1998). *Writing Your Dissertation in Fifteen Minutes a Day*. New York: Henry Holt.
Booth, V. (1993). *Communicating in Science: Writing a Scientific Paper and Speaking at Scientific Meetings*. 2nd edn. Cambridge, UK: Cambridge University Press.
Briscoe, M. H. (1996). *Preparing Scientific Illustrations: A Guide to Better Posters, Presentations, and Publications*. 2nd edn. New York: Springer-Verlag.
Brock, M. H. (1990). *A Researcher's Guide to Scientific and Medical Illustrations*. New York: Springer-Verlag.
Brusau, C. T., Alred, G.J., & Oliu, W.E. (1997). *Handbook of Technical Writing*. 5th edn. New York: St. Martin's Press.
Budavari, S. (ed.) (1998). *The Merck Index: An Encyclopedia of Chemicals and Drugs*. 12th edn. Rahway, NJ: Merck.
Byrne, D. N. (1998). *Publishing Your Medical Research Paper: What They Don't Teach in Medical School*. Baltimore, MD: Williams & Wilkins.
Calisher, C. H. & Fauquet, C. M. (1992). *Stedman's ICTV Virus Words*. Baltimore, MD: Williams & Wilkins.
Campbell, J. B. & Campbell, J. M. (1995). *Mosby's Survival Guide to Medical Abbrevi-*

ations, Acronyms, Prefixes and Suffixes, Symbols and the Greek Alphabet. ed. C. O. Sennet. St. Louis, MO: Mosby-Year Book.

Carosso, R. B. (1986). *Technical Communication.* Belmont, CA: Wadsworth Publishing Co.

Cleveland, W. S. (1994). *The Elements of Graphing Data.* 2nd edn. Boca Raton, FL: CRC Press.

Cooper, H. (1998). *Synthesizing Research.* 3rd edn. Thousand Oaks, CA: Sage.

Council of Biology Editors. (1988). *Illustrating Science: Standards for Publication.* Bethesda, MD: Council of Biology Editors.

Council of Biology Editors (1994). *Scientific Style and Format: The CBE Style Manual for Authors, Editors, and Publishers.* 6th edn. New York: Cambridge University Press.

Covey, S. R. (1989). *The Seven Habits of Highly Effective People.* New York: Simon & Schuster.

Coyle, K. (1997). *Coyle's Information Highway Handbook: A Practical File on the New Information Order.* Chicago, IL: American Library Association.

Crowell, T. L. Jr. (1964). *Index to Modern English.* New York: McGraw-Hill.

Darwin, F. (ed.) (1987). (reprinted 1925). *The Life and Letters of Charles Darwin, Including an Autobiographical Chapter.* New York: Dutton.

Day, R. A. (1996). *Scientific English: A Guide for Scientists and Other Professionals.* 2nd edn. Phoenix, AZ: The Oryx Press.

Day, R. A. (1998). *How to Write and Publish a Scientific Paper.* 5th edn. Phoenix, AZ: The Oryx Press.

de Lacey, G., Record, C., & Wade, J. (1985). How accurate are quotations and references in medical journals? *British Medical Journal,* **291,** 884–6.

DeSousa, L. R., DeSousa, J. S., DeSousa, S. P., & DeSousa, M. C. (1995). *Common Medical Abbreviations.* Albany, NY: Delmar Publishers.

Dixon, B. (1993). Plain words please. *New Scientist,* **137**(1865), 39–40.

Dizon, A. E. & Rosenberg, J. E. (1990). We don't care, Professor Einstein, the Instructions to the Authors specifically said double-spaced. In *Writing for Fishery Journals,* ed. J. Hunter, pp. 65–74. Bethesda, MD: American Fisheries Society.

Dorland's Illustrated Medical Dictionary. (1994). 28th edn. Philadelphia, PA: W. B. Saunders Co.

Dupré, L. (1998). *BUGS in Writing: A Guide to Debugging your Prose,* Rev. edn. Reading, MA: Addison Wesley Longman, Inc.

Eisenberg, A. (1992). *Guide to Technical Editing. Discussion, Dictionary, and Exercises.* New York: Oxford University Press.

Evans, J. T., Nadjari, H. I., & Burchell, S. A. (1990). Quotational and reference accuracy in surgical journals: a continuing peer review problem. *Journal of the American Medical Association,* **263,** 1353–4.

Flower, L. (2000). *Problem Solving Strategies for Writing.* 5th edn. San Diego, CA: Harcourt Brace Jovanovich.

Gilster, P. (1997). *Digital Literacy.* New York: John Wiley & Sons.

Gingras, B. (1987). Simplified English in maintenance manuals. *Technical Communications,* **34**(1), 24–8.

Goldstein, N. (ed.). (1999). *The Associated Press Stylebook and Libel Manual: With Appendices on Photo Captions, Filing the Wire.* 34th edn. New York: Associated Press.

Gould, C. (1998). *Searching Smart on the World Wide Web. Tools and Techniques for Getting Quality Results.* Berkeley, CA: Library Solutions Press.

Gross, D. V. & Sis, R. F. (1980). Scientific writing: The good, the bad, and the ugly. *Journal of Veterinary Medical Education,* **7**(3), 127–30.

Hale, C. (ed.) (1996). *Wired Style: Principles of English Usage in the Digital Age*. San Francisco, CA: Publishers Group West.

Handbook of Current Medical Abbreviations. (1998). 5th edn. Philadelphia, PA: The Charles Press.

Hinchcliff, K. W., Bruce, M. J., Powers, J. D., & Kipp, M. L. (1993). Accuracy of references and quotations in veterinary journals. *Journal of the American Veterinary Medical Association*, **202**(3), 397–400.

Hodges, J. C. (ed.) (1995). *Harbrace College Handbook*. 12th edn. New York: Harcourt Brace Jovanovich.

Hoffman, P. E. (1995). *Netscape and the World Wide Web for Dummies*. Foster City, CA: IDG Books Worldwide, Inc.

Holt, J. G., Kreig, N. R., Sneath, P. H. A., Staley, J. T., & Williams, S. T. (eds.) (1994). *Bergey's Manual of Determinative Bacteriology*. 9th edn. Baltimore, MD: Williams & Wilkins.

Hornby, A. S., Kavanagh, K., & Ashby, M. (1995). *Oxford Advanced Learner's Dictionary of Current English*. 5th edn. New York: Oxford University Press.

Huth, E. J. (1998). *Writing and Publishing in Medicine*. 3rd edn. Baltimore, MD: Williams & Wilkins.

Iles, R. L. (1997). *Guidebook to Better Medical Writing*. Washington, DC: Island Press.

International Association of Business Communicators. (1982). *Without Bias: A Guidebook for Non-discriminatory Communication*. 2nd edn. New York: John Wiley & Sons.

International Botanical Congress. (1988). *International Code of Botanical Nomenclature, adopted by the Fourteenth International Botanical Congress, Berlin, 1987*. Konigstein: Koeltz Scientific Books.

International Code of Zoological Nomenclature.(1999). 4th edn. London: International Trust for Zoological Nomenclature.

International Committee on Taxonomy of Viruses. (1995). *Virus Taxonomy: Classification and Nomenclature of Viruses. Sixth Report of the International Committee on Taxonomy of Viruses*, ed. F. A. Murphy, C. M. Fauquet, D. H. L. Bishop, S. A. Ghabrial, A. W. Jarvis, G. P. Marklli, M. A. Mayo, & M. D. Summers. New York: Springer-Verlag.

International Union of Microbiological Societies. (1992). *International Code of Nomenclature of Bacteria*. 1990 Revision, ed. P. H. A. Sneath, E. F. Lessel, V. B. D. Skerman, H. P. R. Seeliger, & W. A. Clark. Washington, DC: American Society for Microbiology.

Iverson, C. I. (Chair). (1998). *American Medical Association Manual of Style: A Guide for Authors and Editors*. 9th edn. Baltimore, MD: Williams & Wilkins.

Jablonski, S. (ed.) (1998). *Dictionary of Medical Acronyms and Abbreviations*. 3rd edn. Philadelphia, PA: Hanley and Belfus.

Jeffrey, C. (ed.) (1992). *Biological Nomenclature*. 3rd edn. New York: Cambridge University Press.

Lang, T. A. & Secic, M. (1997). *How to Report Statistics in Medicine: Annotated Guidelines for Authors, Editors, and Reviewers. (Medical Writing and Communication)*. Philadelphia, PA: American College of Physicians.

Lawrence, S. (1981). Watching the watchers. *Science News*, **119**, 331–3.

Lederer, R. (1987). *Anguished English*. New York: Dell Publishing.

Leigh, G. J. (1998). *Principles of Chemical Nomenclature: A Guide to IUPAC Recommendations*. Malden, MA: Blackwell Science.

Li, X. & Crane, N. B. (1996). *Electronic Style: A Handbook for Citing Electronic*

Information. 2nd edn. Medford, NJ: Information Today.

Longman Dictionary of American English: A Dictionary for Learners of English. (1997). 2nd edn. Reading, MA: Addison-Wesley.

Lunsford, A. & Connors, R. (1999). *Easy Writer. A Pocket Guide.* New York: St. Martin's Press.

Macdonald-Ross, M. (1977a). Graphics in text. In *Review of Research in Education* No. 5, ed. L. S. Shulman. Itasca, IL: F. E. Peacock.

Macdonald-Ross, M. (1977b). How numbers are shown. *AV Communication Review*, **25**, 359–409.

Mack, K. & Skjei, E. (1979). *Overcoming Writing Blocks.* Los Angeles: J. P. Tarcher. Distributed by St. Martin's Press, New York.

MacNeil, R. (1995). The glorious messiness of English. *Reader's Digest*, Oct. 1995, pp. 151–4.

Maggio, R. (1991). *The Bias-free Word Finder: A Dictionary of Nondiscriminatory Language.* Boston: Beacon Press.

McMillan, V. E. (1997). *Writing Papers in the Biological Sciences.* 2nd edn. New York: St. Martin's Press.

Medical Terms and Abbreviations. (1998). Springhouse, PA: Springhouse Publishing Co.

Nelson, V. (1993). *On Writer's Block.* Boston, MA: Houghton Mifflin Co.

O'Connor, M. (1986). *How to Copyedit Scientific Books and Journals.* Baltimore, MD: Williams & Wilkins.

O'Connor, M. (ed.) (1992). *Writing Successfully in Science.* New York: Chapman & Hall.

Peek, R. P. & Newby, G. B. (eds.) (1996). *Scholarly Publishing. The Electronic Frontier.* Cambridge, MA: The MIT Press.

Peterson, I. (1993). Going for glitz. *Science News*, **144**, 232–3.

Reed, J. G. & Baxter, P. M. (1992). *Library Use: A Handbook for Psychology.* Washington, DC: American Psychological Association.

Rogoff, J. B. & Reiner, S. (1961). Electrodiagnostic apparatus. In *Electrodiagnosis and Electromyography*, 2nd edn. Baltimore: Waverly Press.

Rubens, P. (1992). *Science and Technical Writing: A Manual of Style.* New York: Henry Holt.

Safire, W. (1990). *Fumblerules: A Lighthearted Guide to Grammar and Good Usage.* New York: Doubleday.

Sanderlin, S. (1988). Programming instruction manuals for non-English readers. *Technical Communications*, **35**(2), 96–100.

Schaie, K. W. (1993). Ageist language in psychological research. *American Psychologist*, **48**, 49–51.

Schwartz, M. and the Task Force on Bias-free Language of the Association of American University Presses. (1995). *Guidelines for Bias-free Writing.* Bloomington, IN: Indiana University Press.

Shaw, H. (1993). *Punctuate It Right.* 2nd edn. New York: Harper Collins.

Shortland, M. & Gregory, J. (1991). *Communicating Science: A Handbook.* New York: John Wiley.

Sides, C. H. (1991). *How to Write and Present Technical Information.* 3rd edn. Phoenix, AZ: Oryx Press.

Simmonds, D. & Reynolds, L. (1994). *Data Presentation and Visual Literacy in Medicine and Science.* Stoneham, MA: Butterworth-Heinemann Medical.

Skerman, V. B. D. (ed.) (1989). *Approved Lists of Bacterial Names.* Washington, DC: American Society for Microbiology.

Stedman's Medical Dictionary. (1995). 26th edn. Baltimore, MD: Williams and Wilkins.

Stix, G. (1994). The speed of write. Trends in scientific communication. *Scientific American*, **271**, 106–11.

Strunk, W. Jr. & White, E. B. (2000). *The Elements of Style*, 4th edn. Needham Heights, MA: Allyn & Bacon.

Swanson, E., O'Sean, A. A., & Schleyer, A. T. (1999). *Mathematics into Type* (Updated edn.) Providence, RI: American Mathematical Society.

Turabian, K. L. (1996). *A Manual for Writers of Term Papers, Theses, and Dissertations*, 6th edn. Chicago: University of Chicago Press.

U.S. Trademark Association. (1994). *Trademark Checklist*. New York: U.S. Trademark Association.

USP Dictionary of USAN and International Drug Names. (1998). Rockville, MD: U.S. Pharmacopeial Convention, Inc.

Venolia, J. (1995). *Write Right! A Desktop Digest of Punctuation, Grammar, and Style*. 3rd edn. Berkeley, CA: Ten Speed Press.

Walker, T. J. (1998). The future of scientific journals: free access or pay per view? *American Entomologist*, **44**, 135–8.

Weiss, E. H. (1990). *Writing Remedies: Practical Exercises for Technical Writing*. Phoenix, AZ: Oryx Press.

Wheatley, D. W. & Unwin, A. W. (1972). *The Algorithm Writer's Guide*. London: Longman.

Woodford, F. P. (1968). *Scientific Writing for Graduate Students: A Manual on the Teaching of Scientific Writing*. Bethesda, MD: Council of Biology Editors.

(1999). *How to Teach Scientific Communication*. Bethesda, MD: Council of Biology Editors.

Yang, J. T., Yang, J. N., & Yant, J. T. (1996). *An Outline of Scientific Writing: For Researchers with English as a Foreign Language*. Grandville, MI: World Scientific Publishing Co.

Young, D. S. & Huth, E. J. (1998). *SI Units for Clinical Measurement*. Philadelphia, PA: American College of Physicians.

Zeiger, M. (1991). *Essentials of Writing Biomedical Research Papers*. New York: McGraw-Hill.

Zinsser, W. (1998). *On Writing Well. The Classic Guide to Writing Nonfiction*. 6th edn. New York: Harper.

Appendix 1

Suggested responses to exercises

CHAPTER 1

Exercise 1–1. Message, format, and audience (page 11)

1. Probably not. Simple novelty or extension of a previous record usually is not enough to warrant publication. A case study must change, improve, or enlarge how people think about animal health or disease.
2. The paper your colleague has proposed would have a purpose – to report the case findings – but as a research paper it might not have a message. However, a critical review of case records, coupled with a careful and critical assessment of the literature, might result in a valuable document. A case-series analysis or review article would help busy clinicians get information without laboriously sifting through the primary literature. It would tell investigators where things stand on particular aspects of the disease. And, if well written, it could suggest directions new research should take.
3. Yes, with proper choice of format. Written as a "me-too" series of case histories, the paper will probably be rejected. However, a case-series analysis that would include these data could be a useful contribution.
4. Only one primary research publication is justifiable, because all of the results bear upon your single message. However, this could be supplemented with general articles written for the popular press to reach other target audiences.
5. Psychological researchers, clinicians, psychologists, teachers, school administrators, parents.

CHAPTER 2

Exercise 2–1. Search strategy and Boolean logic (page 32)

1. A, H, J
2. B, E, G
3. D, F
4. A, B, D, E, F, G, H, J
5. F
6. C, I

195

Exercise 2–2. Grammar and style analysis programs (page 49)

1. Twice as many women as men experience migraines.
2. Wanted: Nonsmoking, nondrinking worker to care for cow.
3. I realized that because she was a baboon that grew up wild in the jungle, Wiki had special nutritional needs.
4. The patient with a severe emotional problem was referred to a psychiatrist.
5. Veterinarian Joe Mobbs hoists to its feet a cow injured while giving birth.
6. He wanted a wart removed that had appeared on his left hand about two years ago.
7. Birth control users who smoke are in danger of having retarded children.
8. The woman wants us to operate on the dog's tail again. If it doesn't heal this time, the dog must be humanely killed.

Exercise 2–3. Spellcheckers (page 51)

1. fowl, means, quadrupeds
2. prolific, native
3. congenital
4. prostate
5. dying, algae
6. Danes, Husky
7. coma
8. pistil, its
9. patient, scar
10. words, tip

CHAPTER 3

Exercise 3–1. Organizing ideas (page 60). No response needed.

Exercise 3–2. Title choices (page 69)

1. *Comments:* Overuse of prepositions and trivial phrases takes title over the 10–12 word limit. Two-part title is not accepted by some journals.
   Revision: Verruca [*or* Plantar's Wart] Recurrence after Curative Excision
2. *Comments:* Some editors ban titles that make claims about the findings in the paper.
   Revision: Correlation of Columbine Flower Characteristics and Pollinators
3. *Comments:* Unintended humor arises from careless word choice.
   Revision: Veterinarian Offers Medical Assistance After Panda Mating Fails
4. *Comments:* A century ago, long titles like this one were common. Today they are no longer accepted.
   Revision: Bionomics, Behavior and Taxonomy of Some East Asiatic Crab-ronine Wasps
5. *Comments:* Another overly wordy two-part title, with unintended humor. Titles should not be thinly disguised abstracts.
   Revision: National Health Study on Lung Cancer in Women

CHAPTER 4

Exercise 4–1. Table and figure format choices (page 97)

1. Present the data in a table; some readers might be interested in carrying out their own calculations of relations among the data.
2. Present these data in a table (if exact values are of interest) or by ranges on a map (to show geographical patterns).
3. Present your data in tables or graphs; the relationships are as important as the actual values. Omit the rat photo; it adds no new information.
4. Reading from left to right, the table columns might correspond to the temporal order in which the data were collected, like this: Age–Sex–Complaint–Physical Findings–Laboratory Data–Autopsy Findings.
5. Use the electronmicrograph; it presents new evidence of the bacterial structure. Omit the roentgenogram; no new evidence is provided by a typical example of previously published information.
6. You could present it in a table, a graph, or in the text, but readers will see the point more quickly in a genealogical chart, which is a type of graph.
7. A bar graph would emphasize the difference in mortality, but the same point could be made with equal efficiency in the text. In a lecture or talk, a bar graph might be perfect for added visual emphasis, but readers can scan the text of a paper again if they have missed a point.

CHAPTER FIVE

Exercise 5–1. Revising the first draft (page 103)

A. 10, 1, 6, 2, 5, 3, 9, 11, 7, 8, 4
B. Three copies; read one and annotate changes to be made in margins. Cut and paste a second copy into the new revised order. Save the third copy for possible later reference.

Exercise 5–2. Person and point of view (page 107)

1. As a laboratory technician, you will find that the new procedure is an improvement; you will not need to sterilize the skin. *or* Laboratory technicians will find the new procedure an improvement because they do not need to sterilize the skin.
2. Change "the authors herein" to "we."
3. Change "the authors wish to gratefully acknowledge and thank" to "we thank."
4. The disease is contagious and contamination should be avoided (van der Veen, 1850); cleanliness is essential. *or* Van der Veen (1850) found that the disease is contagious and contamination should be avoided. I agree that cleanliness is essential.
5. I believe that I have discovered a new species of *Australopithecus.*

Exercise 5–3. Readability (page 110)

1. The Haversian system consists of a central canal containing blood vessels and a nerve, surrounded by concentric rings of bony matrix. Between them, scattered tiny spaces called lacunae are filled with bone cells and connected by canaliculi to one another and the central canal. Through these canals the cells are nourished and kept alive.
2. The kidney, a very important organ, has the ability to secrete substances selectively which enables it to maintain proper composition of the blood and other body fluids. Some metabolic end products are injurious if allowed to accumulate.
3. Sex-linked genes explain red–green color blindness in humans. If a woman heterozygous for color blindness marries a normal-visioned man, half of her sons will be color blind. Her normal sons will show no trace of the anomaly and will never transmit it to their children. All of her daughters will have normal vision. However, half of these will be heterozygous for the defect and can have color blind sons. The homozygous daughters will never pass the trait on to either sons or daughters.

Exercise 5–4. Strings of pearls (page 112)

A.

1. mature iron from muscle; iron that is from mature muscle.
2. chronic symptoms of depression; symptoms of chronic depression.
3. excretion of renal lithium; renal excretion of lithium.

B.

1. In their abdomens, the three patients all had tumors that were confirmed to be metastatic and malignant. (Avoid saying "cases" had tumors.)
2. We examined various combinations of immunospecific drugs to see whether any inhibited leukocytes in the peripheral blood of humans. (Avoid saying a study "examines" something.)

Exercise 5–5. Hedging (page 113)

1. These observations suggest a female sex pheromone. (Still marginally incorrect, for an "observation" can't suggest anything, but the meaning would be clear to readers.)
2. Following the outlined procedure might be wise.
3. The study shows an apparent link between cigarette smoking and lung cancer. (Longer but more technically correct: Based on this study, cigarette smoking and lung cancer may be linked.)
4. A cause-and-effect relationship appears likely.
5. The results indicate that the mixture was somewhat saturated with oil. *or* On the basis of these results, the mixture was somewhat saturated with oil.

Exercise 5–6. Revising for brevity (page 118)

A.

1. (Omit entirely.)
2. an uninvestigated possibility is
3. we envision, we feel, etc.
4. critics have stated that
5. (Omit entirely.)

B.

1. The new organism is green, round, 5 × 10 mm, and active (or motile).
2. Twenty to thirty electrophoretic steps usually will be needed.
3. If we meet now about salaries, consensus should be easy to attain.
4. The case load included 15 juveniles and 10 adults. (By definition, juveniles are young and adults are mature; here, "case load" is not jargon, but specialized vocabulary of the field.)
5. Here an alternative is unnecessary. ("In this case" is jargon. If it is not viable, it is not a true alternative; "quite" is unneeded.)
6. Fig. 1. Lateral white cells in abdominal ganglion of live cockroach. Ventral view, anterior at top. (Scale bar, 0.1 mm.)
7. The absence of color was unique.
8. To determine the organism's mobility, state-of-the-art equipment was used.
9. To understand the effects of heat on the organism, we plan to chill it.

CHAPTER 6

Exercise 6–1. Active and passive voice (page 122)

1. One might expect this treatment to be effective. *or* We expect this treatment to be effective.
2. The pathologist had no feed to analyze.
3. Jones and her colleagues inoculated 25 chickens.
4. I traveled to Georgia to collect Lepidoptera.
5. Mark passages A and B for revision.
6. Last night, the campus police reported that two microscopes were stolen.
7. To encourage condom use, the French government has prepared commercials blunt enough to shock even liberal Americans.
8. As a scientific writer, you should state your point clearly at the beginning.
9. This dictionary does not include modern technical words that had no equivalent in ancient spoken Greek and Latin.
10. At the request of the university president, administrative personnel at the Biology Building are studying three incineration systems.

Exercise 6–2. Subject–verb agreement (page 125)

1. The remaining fluid was drawn off, and the kidneys were washed.
2. Due to the small number of test animals used, the data were not statistically significant *or* (if no statistical tests were involved) Due to the small number of test animals used, the data were not meaningful.
3. Extensive karyorrhexis, karyolysis, and hepatocyte degeneration were evident within the centrilobular regions. ("Cellular" is redundant, for hepatocytes couldn't degenerate any other way.)
4. The data indicate that Jones was the first to discover the phenomenon.
5. Not one of the animals was harmed in the course of this study.
6. After a sample was assessed by radiocarbon dating, sections were subjected to potassium–argon analysis.
7. Neither the rats nor the chimpanzee was kept in the laboratory. *or* Neither the chimpanzee nor the rats were kept in the laboratory.
8. Twelve liters of serum were infused into the elephant.

Exercise 6–3. Dangling participles and other misplaced modifiers (page 127)

1. Toward the anterior chamber, a lamination was evident.
2. Using dimethyl sulfoxide, we observed no bacteria.
3. After experimentation, bacteria multiplied.
4. A correlation between the variables was evident with this methodology.
5. With an inverted ocular, intestinal sections can be examined for metazoan parasites.
6. Two of the researchers' stopwatches that had been left leaning against cabinets were badly damaged.
7. For sale: laboratory table with thick legs and large drawers; suitable for researcher.

Exercise 6–4. Comparisons and lists (page 129)

1. The authors' mild pulmonary hypertensive stage was similar to this stage in our study.
2. Group A was more unusual than Group B.
3. The cat recovered better than any of the other cats did.
4. The emergency medical kit contained a bandage, an applicator, a towel, a brush, and a rubber sponge.
5. The fox was heavier than any of the other animals in the study group.
6. Of the two alternatives, this one is the more interesting.

Exercise 6–5. Tense use (page 132)

1. Recent work by Matthews (1980) shows that *Vespula* nests readily in the

laboratory. (Sentence is also correct as it stands, though slightly less smooth.)

2. In our study, bird size increased with width of wooded habitat, as Figure 2 indicates.

3. Beal (1960) also observed (or observes) that size increases with meadow width.

4. In our study we found that there were significantly fewer antibody-producing cells in copper-deficient mice than in copper-supplemented mice (see Fig. 3).

5. Correct as it stands; these results cannot be generalized.

6. Conover and Kynard (1981) reported (*or* report) that sex determination in the Atlantic silverside fish is under the control of both genotype and temperature.

7. Correct as it stands.

8. Correct as it stands.

9. ABSTRACT: The cell-to-cell channels in the insect salivary gland were probed with fluorescent molecules. From the molecular dimensions, a permeation-limiting channel diameter of 16–20 Å was obtained.

10. SUMMARY: Germinal and somatic functions in *Tetrahymena* were found to be performed separately by the micro- and macronuclei, respectively. Cells with haploid micronuclei were mated with diploids to yield monosomic progeny.

Exercise 6–6. Number usage and interpretation (page 140)

1. Three-quarters (75%) of the experimental animals died within 15 hours, but 17 horses (10%) were still alive 45 days later.

2. The chemicals for the experiment cost about $25 and weighed less than 0.2 mg.

3. We calculated that 20,500 cells were affected.

4. The control group recovered more quickly, but the difference was not statistically significant (Chi square test [give probability level here, too, for completeness]).

5. The test plot contained 10 species of grasses, 2 species of legumes, 6 species of trees, and 15 species of cruciferous plants.

CHAPTER 7
Exercise 7–1. Jargon (page 144)

A.

1. easy
2. enough
3. can
4. inhibited
5. in theory, theoretically
6. regularly

B.

1. The "etiology of this disease" means the "study of the cause of this disease." The author intended to say "the cause of this disease."
2. Literally, "histopathology stages" would be stages in the study of the pathology of tissues. The author probably intended to say "histopathological."
3. A "necrology" is a list of persons who have died within a certain time. The author probably meant "necropsy." Avoid saying that the necropsy could "confirm" something; necropsy is the tool which the scientist uses to confirm it.

C.

1. After the operation, the cow ran into a defective electric fence and had to be killed.
2. Position the slide carefully to see the unique shape clearly.
3. I think the drug can ease disease symptoms.

Exercise 7–2. Devil pairs (page 149)

1. like; as
2. whereas; while
3. various; varying
4. effect; effect; effect; affect
5. principle; principal; principle
6. complement; compliment, complement

Exercise 7–3. Which and that (page 150)

1. New fossil evidence indicates that *Cantius,* a primitive primate, had a grasping big toe, which may have figured in the evolution of all modern primates.
2. The use of low weight dextrin should be avoided in these patients. These drugs appear to pass through the damaged endothelium of pulmonary vessels.
3. Occasionally a client will notice a parasite on a fish. The situation is more worrisome to the owner than to the fish.
4. We conclude that during the next year, 10.5 thousand (or 10,500) tons of lead will be emitted into the air in addition to the 90 thousand (or 90,000) tons that are being emitted now.
5. We could not find the proposal that was missing.

Exercise 7–4. Handling language sensitively (page 154)

1. A researcher must be sure to double-check all references.
2. There were 200 Asian participants.

3. Depressed individuals and those with epilepsy reacted to the drug in different ways.
4. The police officer apprehended a person for jaywalking.
5. The ten women in the study included one with cerebral palsy.
6. Breast cancer is one of the oldest diseases known.
7. We need 14 women who are willing to staff the project.

Exercise 7–5. Lazy verbs and warning words (page 157)

A.

1. By early adulthood, more males than females expressed severe symptoms of copper deficiency.
2. Under standard conditions, diazepam inhibited the initial rate of protein phosphorylation (Fig. 1).
3. Soap acts at the cell surface.
4. Stanozolol prolonged appetite.
5. We isolated *A. hydrophila*. (Starting sentence with abbreviation is undesirable.)

B.

1. Physicists hope to solve the question of whether science can harness alternative energy sources.
2. Data were transformed to perform relevant statistical analyses.

CHAPTER 8
Exercise 8–1. Punctuation (page 172)

1. Indicate optimum instrument settings for temperature, humidity, rainfall, and performance.
2. When examined closely, the skeleton bears many bumpy spines that project from the surface of the animal.
3. Class Echinoidea, which includes sea urchins, sand dollars, and heart urchins, is not closely related to class Ascomyceteae.
4. The adults are radially symmetrical, but the larvae are bilateral. It is generally held that this phylum evolved from bilateral ancestors and that radial symmetry arose as an adaptation to a sessile way of life.
5. The clinician asked, "How did the patient die?" The answer was not obvious.
6. The essay, "The Future of Veterinary Medicine," appeared in the early 1960s.

Exercise 8–2. Capitalization (page 175)

1. The Afghan hound ate plaster of Paris.
2. The study sample included 15 Greyhounds, 14 Malamutes, and 10 Spanish Terriers.

3. Adenine and guanine are nucleotides called purines.
4. A person can live normally without the adrenal medullae, but not without the cortices.
5. These bacteria inhabit all biomes in the Northern Hemisphere.
6. *What's So Funny about Science?* by Sidney Harris.
7. Assessment of the Role of Alcohol in the Human Stress Response.
8. A synopsis of the taxonomy of North American and West Indian birds.

Exercise 8–3. Scientific names (page 178)

1. the parasitic wasp, *M. atrata*
2. the dandelion, *Taraxacum officionale,* family Compositae, class Dicotyledonae
3. the honeybee, *Apis mellifera* var. *ligustica*
4. the human malarial parasite, *Plasmodium falciparum* Bignami
5. The starfish *(Asterias)* belongs to the class Asteroidea, phylum Echinodermata, in the section Deuterostomia.

Exercise 8–4. Trade names (page 181)

A.

1. the ammonium hydroxide cleaner, Parson's Sudsy Detergent Ammonia®,[1]
   [1]Armour Dial, Inc., Phoenix, AZ
2. diethylcarbamazine citrate tablets, Decacide®,[1]
   [1]Professional Veterinary Laboratories, Minneapolis, MN

B.

1. After adding water, place the fiberglass cap on the heat-resistant glass pitcher.
2. Please send a photocopy of the figure that shows the sparrow building its nest with facial tissue and transparent tape.
3. Patients should not don in-line skates for at least an hour after receiving botulinum toxin.
4. The abandoned dog survived on canned luncheon meat and petroleum jelly.

Exercise 8–5. Foreign words and phrases (page 183)

1. When acceptable, use the formulas already given in the book, *Official Methods in Microbiology.*
2. For information on the action of green plant pigments, *i.e.,* chlorophyll, *in vivo* see Arnon's article in *Scientific American* and Bassham's book, *The Photosynthesis of Carbon Compounds.*
3. Our experiments cannot identify the underlying biophysical alterations, namely, effects within the membrane itself.
4. Reduced oxygen tension provides the best environment for parasite development *in vitro,* as shown by Udeinya *et al.*

Exercise 8–6. Shortened forms (page 187)

1. Do not use abbreviations (TCGF, SPAFAS) in titles. Do not abbreviate U.S. except as an adjective.
2. Do not use undefined abbreviations in abstracts. Do not abbreviate units of measurement (hrs.) when they are used without numerals.
3. This alphabet soup sentence is annoyingly cryptic.
4. Do not abbreviate units of measurement used without numerals.
5. Abbreviation of state names is inconsistent and that of South Carolina follows neither approved system.

Practicing mixed corrections – a self-test (page 188)

1. *Comments*: Wordy; change numbers to Arabic; use first person.
   Revision: We conclude that these mammalian cells have a limiting diameter of 16–20 Å.
2. *Comments*: Subject–verb disagreement; use of passive could be changed.
   Revision: We studied the inhibitory activity of the various combinations and plotted isobolograms.
3. *Comments*: Wordy, awkward; "at . . . by" construction sounds like location; "increasing" may be interpreted two ways.
   Revision: At the cell surface, EDTA increases cell wall permeability. (Remember not to start a sentence with an abbreviation.)
4. *Comments*: wordy.
   Revision: The pronounced heart lesions were measured.
5. *Comments*: Two meanings possible for "numerous" – many strains, or strains which have many individuals; incorrect use of italics and capitalization. An exception to the usual rule regarding diseases, Chagas is capitalized because it is derived from a proper noun, the name of its describer.
   Revision: Many strains of *T. cruzi* cause Chagas disease.
6. *Comments*: A report of one's current research requires past tense; "irritated" gives sentence an amusing double meaning. (Author probably meant it in the sense of "inflamed," not "annoyed.")
   Revision: Treatment stopped when fish showed signs of physical irritation.
7. *Comments*: Dangling phrase – whose middle legs, those of the wasp or those of the fly? Which does "ventrally" refer to? Preferable not to start sentence with an abbreviation; scientific name needs italics. Progressive provisioner is an acceptable technical term.
   Revision: A progressive provisioner, *S. maculata* carries flies beneath its body with its middle legs.
8. *Comments*: How can a figure be a fish? Does a pond have metacercariae or a gill cavity?
   Revision: Metacercariae (arrow, Fig. 24) were evident in the gill cavity of a cichlid fish found in a Florida pond.
9. *Comments*: Unnecessary words; measurements could be simplified.
   Revision: Mix 1.5 liters dye with 7 liters water.

10. *Comments*: A list in which some items begin with a vowel and some do not requires an article with each; series requires comma before "and." Generic names should be underlined or italicized. Given the information to know the statement was true, pluralization would make the sentence read more smoothly.
    Revision: Fruits in the *Artibeus* diet included an orange, a pear, an apple, and a peach. Fruits in the *Artibeus* diet included oranges, pears, apples, and peaches.
11. *Comments*: Misplaced modifier, sounds like fish have cilia. Generic names should be underlined or italicized.
    Revision: *Ichthyophthirius* is one of the few ciliated parasites infesting fish.
12. *Comments*: "Varying" means changing; author probably meant "various." Use of "the authors" is unclear; if it means authors of this sentence substitute "we."
    Revision: We found amorphous material of various densities.
13. *Comments*: "Equally" and "each" are redundant; "divided" has two meanings.
    Revision: The animals were placed in 5 groups of 22.
14. *Comments*: Sounds like a magician, pulling swabs out of tracheas.
    Revision: With cotton swabs, we obtained tracheal samples.
15. *Comments*: Too much hedging; use present tense for published findings that can be generalized. The qualifiers "many" and "sometimes" (or "at times") both are needed to avoid changing the meaning.
    Revision: Many of their published results indicate that MG organisms sometimes are transmitted poorly.
16. *Comments*: Misplaced phrase – feeds with resolution? Punctuation needed; active tense improves sentence.
    Revision: We used HPLC, a technique with excellent resolution, to analyze aflatoxins in feeds.
17. *Comments*: Hiccups; redundancy; wordiness.
    Revision: A possible cause is aflatoxin entering the bloodstream.
18. *Comments*: Wordy and pretentious.
    Revision: Too much sunlight can burn skin.
19. *Comments*: For a restrictive clause, "that" is preferable; passive, colorless verb; "continual" is used improperly; some redundancy.
    Revision: When it circled, the horse was continuously lame.
20. *Comments*: Restrictive clause should not be set off by commas; rewording would make sentence read more smoothly.
    Revision: The unexercised dogs housed in runs developed no clinical signs of heartworm disease.

Appendix 2

Uniform requirements for manuscripts submitted to biomedical journals*

Updated May 1999

A small group of editors of general medical journals met informally in Vancouver, British Columbia, in 1978 to establish guidelines for the format of manuscripts submitted to their journals. The group became known as the Vancouver Group. Its requirements for manuscripts, including formats for bibliographic references developed by the National Library of Medicine, were first published in 1979. The Vancouver Group expanded and evolved into the International Committee of Medical Journal Editors (ICMJE), which meets annually; gradually it has broadened its concerns.

The committee has produced five editions of the *Uniform Requirements for Manuscripts Submitted to Biomedical Journals*. Over the years, issues have arisen that go beyond manuscript preparation. Some of these issues are now covered in the *Uniform Requirements*; others are addressed in separate statements. Each statement has been published in a scientific journal.

The fifth edition (1997) is an effort to reorganize and reword the fourth edition to increase clarity and address concerns about rights, privacy, descriptions of methods, and other matters. The total content of *Uniform Requirements for Manuscripts Submitted to Biomedical Journals* may be reproduced for educational, not-for-profit purposes with-

* Reproduced from International Committee of Medical Journal Editors, 1997. This document has been published in several journals and is not covered by copyright. It may be copied or reprinted without permission if such use is not for profit. This document is also available online at various Web sites including

<http://www.acponline.org/journals/annals/01jan97/unifreq.htm>

Inquiries and comments should be sent to Kathleen Case at the ICMJE secretariat office, *Annals of Internal Medicine*, American College of Physicians, Independence Mall West, Sixth Street at Race, Philadelphia, PA 19106-1572, USA. Phone: 215-351-2661; fax: 215-351-2644; email: Kathyc@mail.acponline.org

out regard for copyright; the committee encourages distribution of the material.

Journals that agree to use the *Uniform Requirements* (over 500 do so) are asked to cite the 1997 document in their instructions to authors.

It is important to emphasize what these requirements do and do not imply.

First, the *Uniform Requirements* are instructions to authors on how to prepare manuscripts, not to editors on publication style. (But many journals have drawn on them for elements of their publication styles.)

Second, if authors prepare their manuscripts in the style specified in these requirements, editors of the participating journals will not return the manuscripts for changes in style before considering them for publication. In the publishing process, however, the journals may alter accepted manuscripts to conform with details of their publication style.

Third, authors sending manuscripts to a participating journal should not try to prepare them in accordance with the publication style of that journal but should follow the *Uniform Requirements*.

Authors must also follow the *Instructions to Authors* in the journal as to what topics are suitable for that journal and the types of papers that may be submitted – for example, original articles, reviews, or case reports. In addition, the journal's instructions are likely to contain other requirements unique to that journal, such as the number of copies of a manuscript that are required, acceptable languages, length of articles, and approved abbreviations.

Participating journals are expected to state in their *Instructions to Authors* that their requirements are in accordance with the *Uniform Requirements for Manuscripts Submitted to Biomedical Journals* and to cite a published version.

ISSUES TO CONSIDER BEFORE SUBMITTING A MANUSCRIPT

Redundant or duplicate publication

Redundant or duplicate publication is publication of a paper that overlaps substantially with one already published.

Readers of primary source periodicals deserve to be able to trust that what they are reading is original unless there is a clear statement that the article is being republished by the choice of the author and editor. The bases of this position are international copyright laws, ethical conduct, and cost-effective use of resources.

Most journals do not wish to receive papers on work that has already been reported in large part in a published article or is contained in another paper that has been submitted or accepted for publication elsewhere, in print or in electronic media. This policy does not preclude the journal considering a paper that has been rejected by another journal, or a complete report that follows publication of a preliminary report, such as an abstract or poster displayed for colleagues at a professional meeting. Nor does it prevent journals considering a paper that has been presented at a scientific meeting but not published in full or that is being considered for publication in a proceedings or similar format. Press reports of scheduled meetings will not usually be regarded as breaches of this rule, but such reports should not be amplified by additional data or copies of tables and illustrations.

When submitting a paper, the author should always make a full statement to the editor about all submissions and previous reports that might be regarded as redundant or duplicate publication of the same or very similar work. The author should alert the editor if the work includes subjects about which a previous report has been published. Any such work should be referred to and referenced in the new paper. Copies of such material should be included with the submitted paper to help the editor decide how to handle the matter.

If redundant or duplicate publication is attempted or occurs without such notification, authors should expect editorial action to be taken. At the least, prompt rejection of the submitted manuscript should be expected. If the editor was not aware of the violations and the article has already been published, then a notice of redundant or duplicate publication will probably be published with or without the author's explanation or approval.

Preliminary reporting to public media, governmental agencies, or manufacturers, of scientific information described in a paper or a letter to the editor that has been accepted but not yet published violates the policies of many journals. Such reporting may be warranted when the paper or letter describes major therapeutic advances or public health hazards such as serious adverse effects of drugs, vaccines, other biological products, or medicinal devices, or reportable diseases. This reporting should not jeopardize publication, but should be discussed with and agreed upon by the editor in advance.

Acceptable secondary publication

Secondary publication in the same or another language, especially in other countries, is justifiable, and can be beneficial, provided all of the following conditions are met.

1. The authors have received approval from the editors of both journals; the editor concerned with secondary publication must have a photocopy, reprint, or manuscript of the primary version.
2. The priority of the primary publication is respected by a publication interval of at least one week (unless specifically negotiated otherwise by both editors).
3. The paper for secondary publication is intended for a different group of readers; an abbreviated version could be sufficient.
4. The secondary version faithfully reflects the data and interpretations of the primary version.
5. The footnote on the title page of the secondary version informs readers, peers, and documenting agencies that the paper has been published in

whole or in part and states the primary reference. A suitable footnote might read: "This article is based on a study first reported in the [title of journal, with full reference]."

Permission for such secondary publication should be free of charge.

Protection of patients' rights to privacy

Patients have a right to privacy that should not be infringed without informed consent. Identifying information should not be published in written descriptions, photographs, and pedigrees unless the information is essential for scientific purposes and the patient (or parent or guardian) gives written informed consent for publication. Informed consent for this purpose requires that the patient be shown the manuscript to be published.

Identifying details should be omitted if they are not essential, but patient data should never be altered or falsified in an attempt to attain anonymity. Complete anonymity is difficult to achieve, and informed consent should be obtained if there is any doubt. For example, masking the eye region in photographs of patients is inadequate protection of anonymity.

The requirement for informed consent should be included in the journal's instructions for authors. When informed consent has been obtained it should be indicated in the published article.

REQUIREMENTS FOR SUBMISSION OF MANUSCRIPTS

Summary of technical requirements

- Double space all parts of manuscripts.
- Begin each section or component on a new page.
- Review the sequence: title page, abstract and key words, text, acknowledgments, references, tables (each on separate page), legends.
- Illustrations, unmounted prints, should be no larger than 203 × 254 mm (8 × 10 inches).
- Include permission to reproduce previously published material or to use illustrations that may identify human subjects.
- Enclose transfer of copyright and other forms.
- Submit required number of paper copies.
- Keep copies of everything submitted.

Preparation of manuscript

The text of observational and experimental articles is usually (but not necessarily) divided into sections with the headings Introduction, Methods, Results, and Discussion. Long articles may need subheadings within some sections (especially the Results and Discussion sections) to clarify their content. Other types of articles, such as case reports, reviews, and editorials, are likely to need other formats. Authors should consult individual journals for further guidance.

Type or print out the manuscript on white bond paper, 216 × 279 mm (8.5 × 11 inches), or ISO A4 (212 × 297 mm), with margins of at least 25 mm (1 inch). Type or print on only one side of the paper. Use double spacing throughout, including for the title page, abstract, text, acknowledgments, references, individual tables, and legends. Number pages consecutively, beginning with the title page. Put the page number in the upper or lower right-hand corner of each page.

Manuscripts on disks

For papers that are close to final acceptance, some journals require authors to provide a copy in electronic form (on a disk); they may accept a variety of word-processing formats or text (ASCII) files.

When submitting disks, authors should:

1. be certain to include a printout of the version of the article that is on the disk;
2. put only the latest version of the manuscript on the disk;
3. name the file clearly;
4. label the disk with the format of the file and the file name;
5. provide information on the hardware and software used.
6. Authors should consult the journal's instructions to authors for acceptable formats, conventions for naming files, number of copies to be submitted, and other details.

Title page

The title page should carry (1) the title of the article, which should be concise but informative; (2) the name by which each author is known, with his or her highest academic degree(s) and institutional affiliation; (3) the name of the department(s) and institution(s) to which the work should be attributed; (4) disclaimers, if any; (5) the name and address of the author responsible for correspondence about the manuscript; (6) the name and address of the author to whom requests for reprints should be addressed or a statement that reprints will not be available from the authors; (7) source(s) of support in the form of grants, equipment, drugs, or all of these; and (8) a short running head or footline of no more than 40 characters (count letters and spaces) at the foot of the title page.

Authorship

All persons designated as authors should qualify for authorship. Each author should have participated sufficiently in the work to take public responsibility for the content.

Authorship credit should be based only on substantial contributions to (1) conception and design, or analysis and interpretation of data; and to (2) drafting the article or revising it critically for important intellectual content; and on (3) final approval of the version to be published. Conditions (1), (2), and (3) must all be met. Participation solely in the acquisition of funding or the collection of data does not justify authorship. General supervision of the research group is not sufficient for authorship. Any part of an article critical to its main conclusions must be the responsibility of at least one author.

Editors may ask authors to describe what each contributed; this information may be published.

Increasingly, multicenter trials are attributed to a corporate author. All members of the group who are named as authors, either in the authorship position below the title or in a footnote, should fully meet the above criteria for authorship. Group members who do not meet these criteria should be listed, with their permission, in the Acknowledgments or in an appendix (see Acknowledgments).

The order of authorship should be a joint decision of the coauthors. Because the order is assigned in different ways, its meaning cannot be inferred accurately unless it is stated by the authors. Authors may wish to explain the order of authorship in a footnote. In deciding on the order, authors should be aware that many journals limit the number of authors listed in the table of contents and that the U.S. National Library of Medicine (NLM) lists in MEDLINE only the first 24 plus the last author when there are more than 25 authors.

Abstract and keywords

The second page should carry an abstract (of no more than 150 words for unstructured abstracts or 250 words for structured abstracts). The abstract should state the purposes of the study or investigation, basic procedures (selection of study subjects or laboratory animals; observational and analytical methods), main findings (giving specific data and their statistical significance, if possible), and the principal conclusions. It should emphasize new and important aspects of the study or observations.

Below the abstract authors should provide, and identify as such, three to ten keywords or short phrases that will assist indexers in cross-indexing the article and may be published with the abstract. Terms from the Medical Subject Headings (MeSH) list of Index Medicus should be used; if suitable MeSH terms are not yet available for recently introduced terms, present terms may be used.

Introduction

State the purpose of the article and summarize the rationale for the study or observation. Give only strictly pertinent references and do not include data or conclusions from the work being reported.

Methods

Describe your selection of the observational or experimental subjects (patients or laboratory animals, including controls) clearly. Identify the age, sex, and other important characteristics of the subjects. The definition and relevance of race and ethnicity are ambiguous. Authors should be particularly careful about using these categories.

Identify the methods, apparatus (give the manufacturer's name and address in parentheses), and procedures in sufficient detail to allow other workers to reproduce the results. Give references to established methods, including statistical methods (see below); provide references and brief descriptions for methods that have been published but are not well known; describe new or substantially modified methods, give reasons for using them, and evaluate their limitations. Identify precisely all drugs and chemicals used, including generic name(s), dose(s), and route(s) of administration.

Reports of randomized clinical trials should present information on all major study elements, including the protocol (study population, interventions or exposures, outcomes, and the rationale for statistical analysis), assignment of interventions (methods of randomization, concealment of allocation to treatment groups), and the method of masking (blinding).

Authors submitting review manuscripts should include a section describing the methods used for locating, selecting, extracting, and synthesizing data. These methods should also be summarized in the abstract.

Ethics

When reporting experiments on human subjects, indicate whether the procedures followed were in accordance with the ethical standards of the responsible committee on human experimentation (institutional or regional) and with the Helsinki Declaration of 1975, as revised in 1983. Do not use patients' names, initials, or hospital numbers, especially in illustrative material. When reporting experiments on animals, indicate whether the institution's or a national research council's guide for, or any national law on, the care and use of laboratory animals was followed.

Statistics

Describe statistical methods with enough detail to enable a knowledgeable reader with access to the original data to verify the reported results. When possible, quantify findings and present them with appropriate indicators of measurement error or uncertainty (such as confidence intervals). Avoid relying solely on statistical hypothesis testing, such as the use of P values, which fails to convey important quantitative information. Discuss the eligibility of experimental subjects. Give details about randomization. Describe the methods for and success of any blinding of observations. Report complications of treatment. Give numbers of observations. Report losses to observation (such as dropouts from a clinical trial). References for the design of the study and statistical methods should be to standard works when possible (with pages stated) rather than to papers in which the designs or methods were originally reported. Specify any general-use computer programs used.

Put a general description of methods in the Methods section. When data are summarized in the Results section, specify the statistical methods used to analyze them. Restrict tables and figures to those needed to explain the argument of the paper and to assess its support. Use graphs as an alternative to tables with many entries; do not duplicate data in graphs and tables. Avoid nontechnical uses of technical terms in statistics, such as "random" (which implies a randomizing device), "normal," "significant," "correlations," and "sample." Define statistical terms, abbreviations, and most symbols.

Results

Present your results in logical sequence in the text, tables, and illustrations. Do not repeat in the text all the data in the tables or illustrations; emphasize or summarize only important observations.

Discussion

Emphasize the new and important aspects of the study and the conclusions that follow from them. Do not repeat in detail data or other material given in the Introduction or the Results section. Include in the Discussion section the implications of the findings and their limitations, including implications for future research. Relate the observations to other relevant studies.

Link the conclusions with the goals of the study but avoid unqualified statements and conclusions not completely supported by the data. In particular, authors should avoid making statements on economic benefits and costs unless their manuscript includes economic data and analyses. Avoid claiming priority and alluding to work that has not been completed. State new hypotheses when warranted, but clearly label them as such. Recommendations, when appropriate, may be included.

Acknowledgments

At an appropriate place in the article (the title-page footnote or an appendix to the text; see the journal's requirements), one or more statements should specify (1) contributions that need acknowledging but do not justify authorship, such as general support by a departmental chair; (2) acknowledgments of technical help; (3) acknowledgments of financial and material support, which should specify the nature of the support; and (4) relationships that may pose a conflict of interest (see Conflict of Interest).

Persons who have contributed intellectually to the paper but whose contributions do not justify authorship may be named and their function or contribution described-for example, "scientific adviser," "critical review of study proposal," "data collection," or "participation in clinical trial." Such persons must have given their permission to be named. Authors are responsible for obtaining written permission from persons acknowledged by name, because readers may infer their endorsement of the data and conclusions.

Technical help should be acknowledged in a paragraph separate from that acknowledging other contributions.

References

References should be numbered consecutively in the order in which they are first mentioned in the text. Identify references in text, tables, and legends by Arabic numerals in parentheses. References cited only in tables or figure legends should be numbered in accordance with the sequence established by the first identification in the text of the particular table or figure.

Use the style of the examples below, which are based on the formats used by the NLM in *Index Medicus*. The titles of journals should be abbreviated according to the style used in *Index Medicus*. Consult the List of Journals Indexed in *Index Medicus*, published annually as a separate publication by the library and as a list in the January issue of *Index Medicus*. The list can also be obtained through the library's web site (<http://www.nlm.nih.gov>).

Avoid using abstracts as references. References to papers accepted but not yet published should be designated as "in press" or "forthcoming"; authors should obtain written permission to cite such papers as well as verification that they have been accepted for publication. Information from manuscripts submitted but not accepted should be cited in the text as "unpublished observations" with written permission from the source.

Avoid citing a "personal communication" unless it provides essential information not available from a public source, in which case the name of the person and date of communication should be cited in parentheses in the text. For scientific articles, authors should obtain written permission and confirmation of accuracy from the source of a personal communication.

The references must be verified by the author(s) against the original documents.

The *Uniform Requirements* style (the Vancouver style) is based largely on an ANSI standard style adapted by the NLM for its databases. Notes have been added where Vancouver style differs from the style now used by NLM.

Articles in journals

1. Standard journal article

List the first six authors followed by *et al.* (*Note:* NLM now lists up through 25 authors; if there are more than 25 authors, NLM lists the first 24, then the last author, then *et al.*)

Vega KJ, Pina I, Krevsky B. Heart transplantation is associated with an increased risk for pancreatobiliary disease. *Ann Intern Med* 1996 Jun 1;124 (11):980–3.

As an option, if a journal carries continuous pagination throughout a volume (as many medical journals do) the month and issue number may be omitted.

(*Note:* For consistency, the option is used throughout the examples in *Uniform Requirements*. NLM does not use the option.)

Vega KJ, Pina I, Krevsky B. Heart transplantation is associated with an increased risk for pancreatobiliary disease. *Ann Intern Med* 1996;124:980–3.

More than six authors:
Parkin DM, Clayton D, Black RJ, Masuyer E, Friedl HP, Ivanov E, *et al.* Childhood leukaemia in Europe after Chernobyl: 5 year follow-up. *Br J Cancer* 1996;73:1006–12.

2. Organization as author

The Cardiac Society of Australia and New Zealand. Clinical exercise stress testing. Safety and performance guidelines. *Med J Aust* 1996;164:282–4.

3. No author given

Cancer in South Africa [editorial]. *S Afr Med J* 1994;84:15.

4. Article not in English

(*Note:* NLM translates the title to English, encloses the translation in square brackets, and adds an abbreviated language designator.)
Ryder TE, Haukeland EA, Solhaug JH. Bilateral infrapatellar seneruptur hostidligere frisk kvinne. *Tidsskr Nor Laegeforen* 1996;116:41–2.

5. Volume with supplement

Shen HM, Zhang QF. Risk assessment of nickel carcinogenicity and occupational lung cancer. *Environ Health Perspect* 1994;102 Suppl 1:275–82.

6. Issue with supplement

Payne DK, Sullivan MD, Massie MJ. Women's psychological reactions to breast cancer. *Semin Oncol* 1996;23(1 Suppl 2):89–97.

7. Volume with part

Ozben T, Nacitarhan S, Tuncer N. Plasma and urine sialic acid in non-insulin dependent diabetes mellitus. *Ann Clin Biochem* 1995;32(Pt 3):303–6.

8. Issue with part

Poole GH, Mills SM. One hundred consecutive cases of flap lacerations of the leg in ageing patients. *N Z Med J* 1994;107(986 Pt 1):377–8.

9. Issue with no volume

Turan I, Wredmark T, Fellander-Tsai L. Arthroscopic ankle arthrodesis in rheumatoid arthritis. *Clin Orthop* 1995;(320):110–4.

10. No issue or volume

Browell DA, Lennard TW. Immunologic status of the cancer patient and the effects of blood transfusion on antitumor responses. *Curr Opin Gen Surg* 1993:325–33.

11. Pagination in Roman numerals

Fisher GA, Sikic BI. Drug resistance in clinical oncology and hematology. Introduction. *Hematol Oncol Clin North Am* 1995 Apr;9(2):xi–xii.

12. Type of article indicated as needed

Enzensberger W, Fischer PA. Metronome in Parkinson's disease [letter]. *Lancet* 1996;347:1337.
Clement J, De Bock R. Hematological complications of hantavirus nephropathy (HVN) [abstract]. *Kidney Int* 1992;42:1285.

13. Article containing retraction

Garey CE, Schwarzman AL, Rise ML, Seyfried TN. Ceruloplasmin gene defect associated with epilepsy in EL mice [retraction of Garey CE, Schwarzman AL, Rise ML, Seyfried TN. In: *Nat Genet* 1994;6:426–31]. *Nat Genet* 1995;11:104.

14. Article retracted

Liou GI, Wang M, Matragoon S. Precocious IRBP gene expression during mouse development [retracted in *Invest Ophthalmol Vis Sci* 1994;35:3127]. *Invest Ophthalmol Vis Sci* 1994;35:1083–8.

15. Article with published erratum

Hamlin JA, Kahn AM. Herniography in symptomatic patients following inguinal hernia repair [published erratum appears in *West J Med* 1995;162:278]. *West J Med* 1995;162:28–31.

Books and other monographs

(*Note:* Previous Vancouver style incorrectly had a comma rather than a semicolon between the publisher and the date.)

16. Personal author(s)

Ringsven MK, Bond D. *Gerontology and leadership skills for nurses.* 2nd ed. Albany (NY): Delmar Publishers; 1996.

17. Editor(s), compiler(s) as author

Norman IJ, Redfern SJ, editors. *Mental health care for elderly people.* New York: Churchill Livingstone; 1996.

18. Organization as author and publisher

Institute of Medicine (US). *Looking at the future of the Medicaid program.* Washington: The Institute; 1992.

19. Chapter in a book

(*Note:* Previous Vancouver style had a colon rather than a p before pagination.) Phillips SJ, Whisnant JP. Hypertension and stroke. In: Laragh JH, Brenner BM, editors. *Hypertension: pathophysiology, diagnosis, and management.* 2nd ed. New York: Raven Press; 1995. p. 465–78.

20. Conference proceedings

Kimura J, Shibasaki H, editors. Recent advances in clinical neurophysiology. *Proceedings of the 10th International Congress of EMG and Clinical Neurophysiology*; 1995 Oct 15–19; Kyoto, Japan. Amsterdam: Elsevier; 1996.

21. Conference paper

Bengtsson S, Solheim BG. Enforcement of data protection, privacy and security in medical informatics. In: Lun KC, Degoulet P, Piemme TE, Rienhoff O, editors. MEDINFO 92. *Proceedings of the 7th World Congress on Medical Informatics*; 1992 Sep 6–10; Geneva, Switzerland. Amsterdam: North-Holland; 1992. p. 1561–5.

22. Scientific or technical report

Issued by funding/sponsoring agency: Smith P, Golladay K. Payment for durable medical equipment billed during skilled nursing facility stays. Final report. Dallas (TX): Dept. of Health and Human Services (US), Office of Evaluation and Inspections; 1994 Oct. Report No.: HHSIGOEI69200860.

Issued by performing agency: Field MJ, Tranquada RE, Feasley JC, editors. Health services research: work force and educational issues. Washington: National Academy Press; 1995. Contract No.: AHCPR282942008. Sponsored by the Agency for Health Care Policy and Research.

23. Dissertation

Kaplan SJ. Post-hospital home health care: the elderly's access and utilization [dissertation]. St. Louis (MO): Washington Univ.; 1995.

24. Patent

Larsen CE, Trip R, Johnson CR, inventors; Novoste Corporation, assignee. Methods for procedures related to the electrophysiology of the heart. US patent 5,529,067. 1995 Jun 25.

Other published material

25. Newspaper article

Lee G. Hospitalizations tied to ozone pollution: study estimates 50,000 admissions annually. *The Washington Post* 1996 Jun 21;Sect. A:3 (col. 5).

26. Audiovisual material

HIV + /AIDS: the facts and the future [videocassette]. St Louis (MO): Mosby-Year Book; 1995.

27. Legal material

Public law: Preventive Health Amendments of 1993, Pub. L. No. 103-183, 107 Stat. 2226 (Dec. 14, 1993). Unenacted bill: Medical Records Confidentiality Act of 1995, S. 1360, 104th Cong., 1st Sess. (1995).

Code of Federal Regulations: Informed Consent, 42 C.F.R. Sect. 441.257 (1995).

Hearing: Increased Drug Abuse: the Impact on the Nation's Emergency Rooms: Hearings Before the Subcomm. on Human Resources and Intergovernmental Relations of the House Comm. on Government Operations, 103rd Cong., 1st Sess. (May 26, 1993).

28. Map

North Carolina. Tuberculosis rates per 100,000 population, 1990 [demographic map]. Raleigh: North Carolina Dept. of Environment, Health, and Natural Resources, Div. of Epidemiology; 1991.

29. Book of the Bible

The Holy Bible. King James version. Grand Rapids (MI): Zondervan Publishing House; 1995. Ruth 3:1–18.

30. Dictionary and similar references

Stedman's medical dictionary. 26th ed. Baltimore: Williams & Wilkins; 1995. Apraxia; p. 119–20.

31. Classical material

The Winter's Tale: act 5, scene 1, lines 13–16. *The complete works of William Shakespeare.* London: Rex; 1973.

Unpublished material

32. In press

(*Note:* NLM prefers "forthcoming" because not all items will be printed.) Leshner AI. Molecular mechanisms of cocaine addiction. *N Engl J Med.* In press 1996.

Electronic material

33. Journal article in electronic format

Morse SS. Factors in the emergence of infectious diseases. *Emerg Infect Dis* [serial online] 1995 Jan–Mar [cited 1996 Jun 5];1(1):[24 screens]. Available from: URL: http://www.cdc.gov/ncidod/EID/eid.htm

34. Monograph in electronic format

CDI, *clinical dermatology illustrated* [monograph on CD-ROM]. Reeves JRT, Maibach H. CMEA Multimedia Group, producers. 2nd ed. Version 2.0. San Diego: CMEA; 1995.

35. Computer file

Hemodynamics III: the ups and downs of hemodynamics [computer program]. Version 2.2. Orlando (FL): Computerized Educational Systems; 1993.

Tables

Type or print out each table with double spacing on a separate sheet of paper. Do not submit tables as photographs. Number tables consecutively in the order of their first citation in the text and supply a brief title for each. Give each column a short or abbreviated heading. Place explanatory matter in footnotes, not in the heading. Explain in footnotes all nonstandard abbreviations that are used in each table. For footnotes use the following symbols, in this sequence:

*, †, ‡, §, ‖, ¶, **, ††, ‡‡

Identify statistical measures of variations, such as standard deviation and standard error of the mean.

Do not use internal horizontal and vertical rules.

Be sure that each table is cited in the text.

If you use data from another published or unpublished source, obtain permission and acknowledge them fully.

The use of too many tables in relation to the length of the text may produce difficulties in the layout of pages. Examine issues of the journal to which you plan to submit your paper to estimate how many tables can be used per 1000 words of text.

The editor, on accepting a paper, may recommend that additional tables containing important backup data too extensive to publish be deposited with an archival service, such as the National Auxiliary Publication Service in the United States, or made available by the authors. In that event an appropriate statement will be added to the text. Submit such tables for consideration with the paper.

Illustrations (Figures)

Submit the required number of complete sets of figures. Figures should be professionally drawn and photographed; freehand or typewritten lettering is unacceptable. Instead of original drawings, X-ray films, and other material, send sharp, glossy, black-and-white photographic prints, usually 127×173 mm (5×7 inches) but no larger than 203×254 mm (8×10 inches). Letters, numbers, and symbols should be clear and even throughout and of sufficient size that when reduced for publication each item will still be legible. Titles and detailed explanations belong in the legends for illustrations not on the illustrations themselves. Each figure should have a label pasted on its back indicating the number of the figure, author's name, and top of the figure. Do not write on the back of figures or scratch or mar them by using paper clips. Do not bend figures or mount them on cardboard.

Photomicrographs should have internal scale markers. Symbols, arrows, or letters used in photomicrographs should contrast with the background.

If photographs of people are used, either the subjects must not be identifiable or their pictures must be accompanied by written permission to use the photograph (see **Protection of patients' rights to privacy**).

Figures should be numbered consecutively according to the order in which they have been first cited in the text. If a figure has been published, acknowledge the original source and submit written permission from the copyright holder to reproduce the material. Permission is required irrespective of authorship or publisher except for documents in the public domain.

For illustrations in color, ascertain whether the journal requires color negatives, positive transparencies, or color prints. Accompanying drawings marked to indicate the region to be reproduced may be useful to the editor. Some journals publish illustrations in color only if the author pays for the extra cost.

Legends for illustrations

Type or print out legends for illustrations using double spacing, starting on a separate page, with Arabic numerals corresponding to the illustrations. When symbols, arrows, numbers, or letters are used to identify parts of the illustrations, identify and explain each one clearly in the legend. Explain the internal scale and identify the method of staining in photomicrographs.

Units of measurement

Measurements of length, height, weight, and volume should be reported in metric units (meter, kilogram, or liter) or their decimal multiples.

Temperatures should be given in degrees Celsius. Blood pressures should be given in millimeters of mercury.

All hematologic and clinical chemistry measurements should be reported in the metric system in terms of the International System of Units (SI). Editors may request that alternative or non-SI units be added by the authors before publication.

Abbreviations and symbols

Use only standard abbreviations. Avoid abbreviations in the title and abstract. The full term for which an abbreviation stands should precede its first use in the text unless it is a standard unit of measurement.

SENDING THE MANUSCRIPT TO THE JOURNAL

Send the required number of copies of the manuscript in a heavy-paper envelope, enclosing the copies and figures in cardboard, if necessary, to prevent the photographs from being bent. Place photographs and transparencies in a separate heavy-paper envelope.

Manuscripts must be accompanied by a covering letter signed by all coauthors. This must include (1) information on prior or duplicate publication or submission elsewhere of any part of the work as defined earlier in this document; (2) a statement of financial or other relationships that might lead to a conflict of interest (see below); (3) a statement that the manuscript has been read and approved by all the authors, that the requirements for authorship as stated earlier in this document have been met, and that each author believes that the manuscript represents honest work; and (4) the name, address, and telephone number of the corresponding author, who is responsible for communicating with the other authors about revisions and final approval of the proofs. The letter should give any additional information that may be helpful to the editor, such as the type of article in the particular journal that the manuscript represents and whether the author(s) would be willing to meet the cost of reproducing color illustrations.

The manuscript must be accompanied by copies of any permissions to reproduce published material, to use illustrations or report information about identifiable people, or to name people for their contributions.

SEPARATE STATEMENTS
Definition of a peer-reviewed journal

A peer-reviewed journal is one that has submitted most of its published articles for review by experts who are not part of the editorial staff. The number and kind of manuscripts sent for review, the number of reviewers, the reviewing procedures, and the use made of the reviewers' opinions may vary, and therefore each journal should publicly disclose its policies in its *Instructions to Authors* for the benefit of readers and potential authors.

Editorial freedom and integrity

Owners and editors of medical journals have a common endeavor – the publication of a reliable and readable journal, produced with due respect for the stated aims of the journal and for costs. The functions of owners and editors, however, are different. Owners have the right to appoint and dismiss editors and to make important business decisions in which editors should be involved to the fullest extent possible. Editors must have full authority for determining the editorial content of the journal. This concept of editorial freedom should be resolutely defended by editors even to the extent of their placing their positions at stake. To secure this freedom in practice, the editor should have direct access to the highest level of ownership, not only to a delegated manager.

Editors of medical journals should have a contract that clearly states the editor's rights and duties in addition to the general terms of the appointment and that defines mechanisms for resolving conflict.

An independent editorial advisory board may be useful in helping the editor establish and maintain editorial policy.

All editors and editors' organizations have the obligation to support the concept of editorial freedom and to draw major transgressions of such freedom to the attention of the international medical community.

Conflict of interest

Conflict of interest for a given manuscript exists when a participant in the peer review and publication process – author, reviewer, and editor – has ties to activities that could inappropriately influence his or her judgment, whether or not judgment is in fact affected. Financial relationships with industry (for example, through employment, consultancies, stock ownership, honoraria, expert testimony), either directly or through immediate family, are usually considered to be the most important conflicts of interest. However, conflicts can occur for other reasons, such as personal relationships, academic competition, and intellectual passion.

Public trust in the peer review process and the credibility of published articles depend in part on how well conflict of interest is handled during writing, peer review, and editorial decision making. Bias can often be identified and eliminated by careful attention to the scientific methods and conclusions of the work.

Financial relationships and their effects are less easily detected than other conflicts of interest. Participants in peer review and publication should disclose their conflicting interests, and the information should be made available so that others can judge their effects for themselves. Because readers may be less able to detect bias in review articles and editorials than in reports of original research, some journals do not accept reviews and editorials from authors with a conflict of interest.

Authors

When they submit a manuscript, whether an article or a letter, authors are responsible for recognizing and disclosing financial and other conflicts of interest that might bias their work. They should acknowledge in the manuscript all financial support for the work and other financial or personal connections to the work.

Reviewers

External peer reviewers should disclose to editors any conflicts of interest that could bias their opinions of the manuscript, and they should disqualify themselves from reviewing specific manuscripts if they believe it to be appropriate. The editors must be made aware of reviewers' conflicts of interest to interpret the reviews and judge for themselves whether the reviewer should be disqualified. Reviewers should not use knowledge of the work, before its publication, to further their own interests.

Editors and staff

Editors who make final decisions about manuscripts should have no personal financial involvement in any of the issues they might judge. Other members of the editorial staff, if they participate in editorial decisions, should provide editors with a current description of their financial interests (as they might relate to editorial judgments) and disqualify themselves from any decisions where they have a conflict of interest. Published articles and letters should include a description of all financial support and any conflict of interest that, in the editors' judgment, readers should know about. Editorial staff should not use the information gained through working with manuscripts for private gain.

Project-specific industry support for research

Authors

Scientists have an ethical obligation to submit creditable research results for publication. Moreover, as the persons directly responsible for their work, scientists should not enter into agreements that interfere with their control over the decision to publish the papers they write.

When they submit a manuscript, whether an article or a letter, authors are responsible for recognizing and disclosing financial and other conflicts of interest that might bias their work. They should acknowledge in the manuscript all financial support for their work and other financial or personal connections to the work.

Editors and staff

Editors who make final decisions about manuscripts should have no personal financial involvement in any of the issues they might judge. Other members of the editorial staff, if they participate in editorial decisions, should provide editors with a current description of their financial interests (as they might relate to editorial judgments) and disqualify themselves from any decisions where they have a conflict of interest. Published articles and letters should include a description of all financial support and any conflict of interest that, in the editors' judgment, readers should know about. Editorial staff should not use the information gained through working with manuscripts for private gain.

Editors should require authors to describe the role of outside sources of project support, if any, in study design; in the collection, analysis and interpretation of data; and in the writing of the report. If the supporting source had no such involvement, the authors should so state. Because the biases potentially introduced by the direct involvement of supporting agencies in research are analogous to methodological biases of other sorts (e.g., study design, statistical and psychological factors), the type and degree of involvement of the supporting agency should be described in the Methods section. Editors should also require disclosure of whether or not the supporting agency controlled or influenced the decision to submit the final manuscript for publication.

Corrections, retractions, and "expressions of concern" about research findings

Editors must assume initially that authors are reporting work based on honest observations. Nevertheless, two types of difficulty may arise.

First, errors may be noted in published articles that require the publication of a correction or erratum of part of the work. It is conceivable that an error could be so serious as to vitiate the entire body of the work, but this is unlikely and should be handled by editors and authors on an individual basis. Such an error should not be confused with inadequacies exposed by the emergence of new scientific information in the normal course of research. The latter require no corrections or withdrawals.

The second type of difficulty is scientific fraud. If substantial doubts arise about the honesty of work, either submitted or published, it is the editor's responsibility to ensure that the question is appropriately pursued (including possible consultation with the authors). However, it is not the task of editors to conduct a full investigation or to make a determination; that responsibility lies with the institution where the work was done or with the funding agency. The editor should be promptly informed of the final decision, and if a fraudulent paper has been published, the journal must print a retraction. If this method of investigation does not result in a satisfactory conclusion, the editor may choose to publish an expression of concern with an explanation.

The retraction or expression of concern, so labeled, should appear on a numbered page in a prominent section of the journal, be listed in the contents page, and include in its heading the title of the original article. It should not simply be a letter to the editor. Ideally, the first author should be the same in the retraction as in the article, although under certain circumstances the editor may accept retractions by other responsible people. The text of the retraction should explain why the article is being retracted and include a bibliographic reference to it.

The validity of previous work by the author of a fraudulent paper cannot be assumed. Editors may ask the author's institution to assure them of the validity of earlier work published in their journals or to retract it. If this is not done they may choose to publish an announcement to the effect that the validity of previously published work is not assured.

Confidentiality

Manuscripts should be reviewed with due respect for authors' confidentiality. In submitting their manuscripts for review, authors entrust editors with the results of their scientific work and creative effort, on which their reputation and career may depend. Authors' rights may be violated by disclosure of the confidential details of the review of their manuscript. Reviewers also have rights to confidentiality, which must be respected by the editor. Confidentiality may have to be breached if dishonesty or fraud is alleged but otherwise must be honored.

Editors should not disclose information about manuscripts (including their receipt, their content, their status in the reviewing process, their criticism by reviewers, or their ultimate fate) to anyone other than the authors themselves and reviewers.

Editors should make clear to their reviewers that manuscripts sent for review are privileged communications and are the private property of the authors. Therefore, reviewers and members of the editorial staff should respect the authors' rights by not publicly discussing the authors' work or appropriating their ideas before the manuscript is published. Reviewers should not be allowed to make copies of the manuscript for their files and should be prohibited from sharing it with others, except with the permission of the editor. Editors should not keep copies of rejected manuscripts.

Opinions differ on whether reviewers should remain anonymous. Some editors require their reviewers to sign the comments returned to authors, but most either request that reviewers' comments not be signed or leave the choice to the reviewer. When comments are not signed, the reviewers' identity must not be revealed to the author or anyone else.

Some journals publish reviewers' comments with the manuscript. No such procedure should be adopted without the consent of the authors and reviewers. However, reviewers' comments may be sent to other reviewers of the same manuscript, and reviewers may be notified of the editor's decision.

Medical journals and the popular media

The public's interest in news of medical research has led the popular media to compete vigorously to get information about research as soon as possible. Researchers and institutions sometimes encourage the reporting of research in the popular media before full publication in a scientific journal by holding a press conference or giving interviews.

The public is entitled to important medical information without unreasonable delay, and editors have a responsibility to play their part in this process. Doctors, however, need to have reports available in full detail before they can advise their patients about the reports' conclusions. In addition, media reports of scientific research before the work has been peer reviewed and fully published may lead to the dissemination of inaccurate or premature conclusions.

Editors may find the following recommendations useful as they seek to establish policies on these issues.

1. Editors can foster the orderly transmission of medical information from researchers, through peer-reviewed journals, to the public. This can be accomplished by an agreement with authors that they will not publicize their work while their manuscript is under consideration or awaiting publication and an agreement with the media that they will not release stories before publication in the journal, in return for which the journal will cooperate with them in preparing accurate stories (see below).

2. Very little medical research has such clear and urgently important clinical implications for the public's health that the news must be released before full publication in a journal. In such exceptional circumstances, however, appropriate authorities responsible for public health should make the decision and should be responsible for the advance dissemination of information to physicians and the media. If the author and the appropriate authorities wish to have a manuscript considered by a particular journal, the editor should be consulted before any public release. If editors accept the need for immediate release, they should waive their policies limiting prepublication publicity.

3. Policies designed to limit prepublication publicity should not apply to accounts in the media of presentations at scientific meetings or to the abstracts from these meetings (see **Redundant or duplicate publication**). Researchers who present their work at a scientific meeting should feel free to discuss their presentations with reporters, but they should be discouraged from offering more detail about their study than was presented in their talk.

4. When an article is soon to be published, editors may wish to help the media prepare accurate reports by providing news releases, answering questions, supplying advance copies of the journal, or referring reporters to the appropriate experts. This assistance should be contingent on the media's cooperation in timing their release of stories to coincide with the publication of the article.

Advertising

Most medical journals carry advertising, which generates income for their publishers, but advertising must not be allowed to influence editorial decisions. Editors must have full responsibility for advertising policy. Readers should be able to distinguish readily between advertising and editorial material. The juxtaposition of editorial and advertising material on the same products or subjects should be avoided, and advertising should not be sold on the condition that it will appear in the same issue as a particular article. Journals should not be dominated by advertising, but editors should be careful about publishing advertisements from only one or two advertisers as readers may perceive that the editor has been influenced by these advertisers.

Journals should not carry advertisements for products that have proved to be seriously harmful to health – for example, tobacco. Editors should ensure that existing standards for advertisements are enforced or develop their own standards. Finally, editors should consider all criticisms of advertisements for publication.

Supplements

Supplements are collections of papers that deal with related issues or topics, are published as a separate issue of the journal or as a second part of a regular issue, and are usually funded by sources other than the journal's publisher. Supplements can serve useful purposes: education, exchange of research information, ease of access to focused content, and improved cooperation between academic and corporate entities. Because of the funding sources, the content of supplements can reflect biases in choice of topics and viewpoints. Editors should therefore consider the following principles.

1. The journal editor must take full responsibility for the policies, practices, and content of supplements. The journal editor must approve the appointment of any editor of the supplement and retain the authority to reject papers.
2. The sources of funding for the research, meeting, and publication should be clearly stated and prominently located in the supplement, preferably on each page. Whenever possible, funding should come from more than one sponsor.
3. Advertising in supplements should follow the same policies as those of the rest of the journal.
4. Editors should enable readers to distinguish readily between ordinary editorial pages and supplement pages.
5. Editing by the funding organization should not be permitted.
6. Journal editors and supplement editors should not accept personal favors or excessive compensation from sponsors of supplements.
7. Secondary publication in supplements should be clearly identified by the citation of the original paper. Redundant publication should be avoided.

The role of the correspondence column

All biomedical journals should have a section carrying comments, questions, or criticisms about articles they have published and where the original authors can respond. Usually, but not necessarily, this may take the form of a correspondence column. The lack of such a section denies readers the possibility of responding to articles in the same journal that published the original work.

Competing manuscripts based on the same study

Editors may receive manuscripts from different authors offering competing interpretations of the same study. They have to decide whether to review competing manuscripts submitted to them more or less simultaneously by different groups or authors, or they may be asked to consider one such manuscript while a competing manuscript has been or will be submitted to another journal. Setting aside the unresolved question of ownership of data, we discuss here what editors ought to do when confronted with the submission of competing manuscripts based on the same study.

Two kinds of multiple submissions are considered: submissions by coworkers who disagree on the analysis and interpretation of their study, and submissions by coworkers who disagree on what the facts are and which data should be reported.

The following general observations may help editors and others dealing with this problem.

Differences in analysis or interpretation

Journals would not normally wish to publish separate articles by contending members of a research team who have differing analyses and interpretations of the data, and submission of such manuscripts should be discouraged. If coworkers cannot resolve their differences in interpretation before submitting a manuscript, they should consider submitting one manuscript containing multiple interpretations and calling their dispute to the attention of the editor so that reviewers can focus on the problem. One of the important functions of peer review is to evaluate the authors' analysis and interpretation and to suggest appropriate changes to the conclusions before publication. Alternatively, after the disputed version is published, editors may wish to consider a letter to the editor or a second manuscript from the dissenting authors. Multiple submissions present editors with a dilemma. Publication of contending manuscripts to air authors' disputes may waste journal space and confuse readers. On the other hand, if editors knowingly publish a manuscript written by only some of the collaborating team, they could be denying the rest of the team their legitimate coauthorship rights.

Differences in reported methods or results

Workers sometimes differ in their opinions about what was actually done or observed and which data ought to be reported. Peer review cannot be expected to resolve this problem. Editors should decline further consideration of such multiple submissions until the problem is settled. Furthermore, if there are allegations of dishonesty or fraud, editors should inform the appropriate authorities.

The cases described above should be distinguished from instances in which independent, noncollaborating authors submit separate manuscripts based on different analyses of data that are publicly available. In this circumstance, editorial consideration of multiple submissions may be justified, and there may even be a good reason for publishing more than one manuscript because different analytical approaches may be complementary and equally valid.

Index

Key: *T*, table; *F*, figure; *Ex*, exercise